Rapid Infection Control Nursing

T0258273

Rapid Infection Control Nursing

Shona Ross MPH, BSc, RN
Clinical Nurse Specialist, Infection Prevention and Control
Kingston Hospital
Kingston Upon Thames
UK

and

Sarah Furrows MBBS, MSc, MRCP, FRCPath
Consultant Microbiologist and Infection Control Doctor
Kingston Hospital
Kingston Upon Thames
UK

WILEY Blackwell

This edition first published 2014 © 2014 by John Wiley & Sons, Ltd

Registered Office
John Wiley & Sons, Ltd, The Atrium, Southern Gate, Chichester, West Sussex, PO19 8SQ, UK

Editorial Offices
9600 Garsington Road, Oxford, OX4 2DQ, UK
The Atrium, Southern Gate, Chichester, West Sussex, PO19 8SQ, UK
111 River Street, Hoboken, NJ 07030–5774, USA

For details of our global editorial offices, for customer services and for information about how to apply for permission to reuse the copyright material in this book please see our website at www.wiley.com/wiley-blackwell

The right of the authors to be identified as the authors of this work has been asserted in accordance with the UK Copyright, Designs and Patents Act 1988.

All rights reserved. No part of this publication may be reproduced, stored in a retrieval system, or transmitted, in any form or by any means, electronic, mechanical, photocopying, recording or otherwise, except as permitted by the UK Copyright, Designs and Patents Act 1988, without the prior permission of the publisher.

Designations used by companies to distinguish their products are often claimed as trademarks. All brand names and product names used in this book are trade names, service marks, trademarks or registered trademarks of their respective owners. The publisher is not associated with any product or vendor mentioned in this book. It is sold on the understanding that the publisher is not engaged in rendering professional services. If professional advice or other expert assistance is required, the services of a competent professional should be sought.

The contents of this work are intended to further general scientific research, understanding, and discussion only and are not intended and should not be relied upon as recommending or promoting a specific method, diagnosis, or treatment by health science practitioners for any particular patient. The publisher and the author make no representations or warranties with respect to the accuracy or completeness of the contents of this work and specifically disclaim all warranties, including without limitation any implied warranties of fitness for a particular purpose. In view of ongoing research, equipment modifications, changes in governmental regulations, and the constant flow of information relating to the use of medicines, equipment, and devices, the reader is urged to review and evaluate the information provided in the package insert or instructions for each medicine, equipment, or device for, among other things, any changes in the instructions or indication of usage and for added warnings and precautions. Readers should consult with a specialist where appropriate. The fact that an organization or Website is referred to in this work as a citation and/or a potential source of further information does not mean that the author or the publisher endorses the information the organization or Website may provide or recommendations it may make. Further, readers should be aware that Internet Websites listed in this work may have changed or disappeared between when this work was written and when it is read. No warranty may be created or extended by any promotional statements for this work. Neither the publisher nor the author shall be liable for any damages arising herefrom.

Library of Congress Cataloging-in-Publication Data

Ross, Shona, author.
  Rapid infection control nursing / Shona Ross and Sarah Furrows.
    p. ; cm. – (Rapid series)
  Includes bibliographical references and index.
  ISBN 978-1-118-34246-6 (paper : alk. paper)
  I. Furrows, Sarah, author. II. Title. III. Series: Rapid series.
  [DNLM: 1. Cross Infection–nursing–Handbooks.   2. Cross Infection–prevention & control–Handbooks.
3. Infection Control–Handbooks. WY 49]
  RC112
  362.1969–dc23
                                        2013026511
A catalogue record for this book is available from the British Library.

Wiley also publishes its books in a variety of electronic formats. Some content that appears in print may not be available in electronic books.

Cover image: 'Washing hand with clean water' © defun/iStock
Cover design by Fortiori Design

Set in 7.5/9.5pt Frutiger by SPi Publisher Services, Pondicherry, India

1   2014

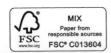

Contents

Acknowledgements

Thanks to our friends and family for putting up with us while this book was written! Thanks also to our colleagues, especially Fran Brooke-Pearce, Victoria Wells and Dr Phil Rice, for their invaluable input.

Foreword

We have come a long way in our quest to reduce healthcare-associated infections since 2005. Major improvements have been made in the way we protect our patients from infection, with once unimaginable reductions being achieved in MRSA bacteraemia and *Clostridium difficile*. Patients once fearful of entering a hospital for fear of acquiring a 'super-bug' now have confidence that hospitals are much cleaner and safer. An important element of this success was making the shift from infection issues being the domain of the infection control team to making infection prevention everyone's responsibility and getting staff to believe that they had a role to play. There was also recognition that there was variation in staff knowledge of effective infection prevention control, and therefore a need to reinforce the components of good practice and be assured that all staff caring for patients had the required knowledge and competence.

When I initially embarked on leading the national HCAI programme, as a non-specialist I had to ask questions, unpick the jargon and 'technical speak' and attempt to simplify the language used around infection. This book does this and would have been hugely helpful to me in 2005.

Good hand hygiene, prompt isolation, prudent antimicrobial prescribing, high standards of cleanliness and aseptic technique when inserting and caring for invasive devices remain the linchpin of good infection prevention and control and consistent reliable application of these principles have underpinned the success to date. That said, there are still other infections and still areas that require further focus, new staff commencing work in many care settings and a need to regularly refresh knowledge. Therefore this book comes at a good time. It does not assume knowledge and explains what staff need to do to protect patients and prevent infection in a simple, clear and comprehensive manner. The book also provides very helpful information on those infections that currently do not feature so prominently in the public eye but are equally important.

We know that the challenge to reduce infection is relentless and it is important that we never become complacent or reduce our focus because of the progress we have made in the last five years. Following the advice in this book will keep us on the right path and ensure we continue on our journey to achieving a zero tolerance to preventable infection. After all, our patients and their families deserve no less.

Professor Janice Stevens CBE, MA, RGN

1 Introduction

This book covers the standard principles of infection prevention and control, which should be adhered to at all times, and provides concise guidance for immediate infection control management of patients with a range of infections. The book is not intended to replace more comprehensive texts, but should be used in conjunction with them.

The authors would urge the reader to adhere to guidance contained within the Infection Prevention and Control Manual in their place of work at all times, as locally developed guidance may differ from what is written here.

The idea for this book came from the questions asked by nurses and other healthcare professionals during training sessions, ward rounds and phone calls received by the infection control team from nurses seeking advice on how to care for a patient with a specific infection.

Hospital infection control policies are not always immediately accessible to staff who are busy caring for patients and, even when policies are accessed, staff often wish to discuss the advice given just to check that they are doing the right thing. Clinical governance arrangements dictate that policies must be formatted in a certain way, which does not enhance their readability or improve the accessibility of the information sought by the nurse with the infected patient in front of her/him. In some instances the language used can be obstructive and unhelpful, with acronyms and jargon used, which are not necessarily understood by the intended audience.

This book was written by an infection control nurse and an infection control doctor with the aim of making it easier for ward nurses to get infection control right. The book is set out in such a way that the information required about immediate infection prevention and control measures is given first and further information is given later. There is no jargon; abbreviations are limited and fully explained where used and every attempt has been made to demystify some of the language and terminology commonly used within the realms of infection control.

Rapid Infection Control Nursing, First Edition. Shona Ross and Sarah Furrows.
© 2014 John Wiley & Sons, Ltd. Published 2014 by John Wiley & Sons, Ltd.

2   The Essentials

The chain of infection

Transmission of infection is a complex process involving a number of factors referred to as 'the chain of infection' (shown in Figure 1).

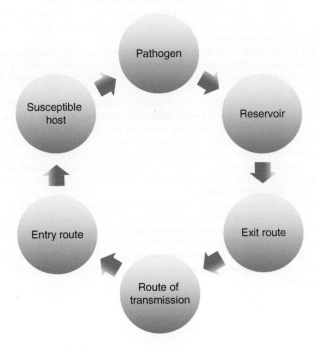

Figure 1   The chain of infection

In order for transmission of infection to occur all of the following elements must be present:

- Presence of an infectious agent (pathogen), e.g. MRSA, *Clostridium difficile*, influenza, etc.
- A reservoir where the organism can live and thrive and replicate, e.g. soil, water, animals, people, inanimate objects (the environment).

Rapid Infection Control Nursing, First Edition. Shona Ross and Sarah Furrows.
© 2014 John Wiley & Sons, Ltd. Published 2014 by John Wiley & Sons, Ltd.

- An exit route for the pathogen to escape its reservoir: urine, vomit, sputum, blood, faeces and the airborne route.
- A transmission route:
  - direct contact: kissing, touching, biting, sexual intercourse, droplet spread into the mouth, eyes and nose during coughing, sneezing, singing and talking; faecal–oral route via ingestion of faeces;
  - indirect contact: via contaminated bedding, clothing, crockery, cutlery, surgical instruments, dressings, water, food and toys; via blood and body fluids; via the hands of healthcare workers; via vectors such as biting or crawling insects; faecal–oral route via contaminated food or objects, e.g. toilet flush handles and toys;
  - airborne spread where an aerosol containing the pathogen is inhaled.
- An entry route: inoculation, ingestion, sexual contact, vertical transmission, inhalation, vector-borne, e.g. malaria.
- A susceptible host – many people are susceptible to infection for a variety of reasons, for example:
  - those with a weakened immune system caused by advancing age or immaturity, medication, disease;
  - those whose natural defences are compromised through surgery, interventions and disease; the presence of wounds, non-intact skin, indwelling medical devices such as urinary catheters, intravenous cannula, etc.

The chain of infection can be broken by using the standard principles of infection prevention and control.

Standard principles of infection prevention and control

These principles were originally referred to as 'universal precautions' and are often referred to as 'standard precautions'.

To break the chain of infection the standard principles of infection control should be applied, which are:

1. Hand hygiene.
2. Correct use of personal protective equipment (gloves, aprons, visors and masks).
3. Control of the environment, which incorporates:
   o decontamination (of healthcare equipment and the healthcare environment; management of blood and body fluid spillages);
   o isolation and cohorting;
   o respiratory hygiene;
   o safe management of sharps and splash injuries;
   o safe sharps practice;
   o safe disposal of clinical waste;
   o safe handling of linen and laundry.

The aseptic non-touch technique is included here, as it is essential for infection prevention and control.

Hand hygiene

Washing the hands is the most effective way to prevent the spread of infection. This section is broken down into two subsections: the first covers when to wash the hands and the technique for doing so effectively; the second section discusses hand hygiene equipment, including soap, nailbrushes and hand washbasins.

When and how to clean the hands

WHEN   Hands should be cleaned at the 'five moments for hand hygiene':

1. Before touching a patient.
2. Before a clean/aseptic procedure.
3. After exposure to blood/body fluids.
4. After touching a patient.
5. After touching a patient's surroundings.

More broadly speaking, this includes:

- Before and after handling invasive devices (moments 1, 2 and 3).
- Before and after dressing wounds (moments 1, 2 and 3).
- Before and after contact with immunocompromised patients (moments 1 and 4).
- After contact with equipment contaminated with blood/body fluid (moment 3).
- After contact with blood/body fluid (moment 3).
- After handling used laundry and clinical waste (moment 3).
- After glove removal (moment 3).
- Before leaving the clinical area (moments 4 and 5).
- After using the toilet (not specific to healthcare, but essential).
- Before and after handling food/drink (not specific to healthcare, but essential).

HOW   Using the six-step technique for hand washing (below) described by Ayliffe *et al.* (1978) should take approximately 15–20 seconds and allows all surfaces of the hands to be cleaned effectively. The mechanical action of rubbing the hands together is important in hand washing to dislodge bacteria from the skin's surface.

Hands should be wet before soap is applied in order to get a better lather and spread of the soap and to avoid the irritation that can occur when soap is applied directly to the skin, repeatedly.

1. Rub hands together palm to palm.
2. Rub hands together, palm to palm with fingers interlaced.
3. Rub left hand over right hand with palm of left hand rubbing back of right hand, with fingers interlaced, and then right hand over left hand with palm of right hand rubbing back of left hand, with fingers interlaced.
4. Rub fingertips of left hand into right palm and fingertips of right hand into left palm.
5. Rub hands together with backs of fingers to opposing palms.
6. Grip thumb of left hand with right hand and rub in a rotational manner and then repeat on the other side.

The hands should then be rinsed and dried thoroughly.

Surgical scrubbing/rubbing

Surgical scrubbing/rubbing involves using the six-step technique described above to wash the hands, including the forearms. An antibacterial soap is used and the process takes around two minutes.

- Surgical scrubbing/rubbing is essential before donning sterile theatre gowns, gloves, etc.
- All hand and wrist jewellery must be removed.
- Nailbrushes should not be used but nail picks can be used if the nails appear dirty.

Hand hygiene equipment

SOAP AND WATER   Plain liquid soap and water are adequate for hand washing for the majority of clinical care activities – the technique used to clean the hands is more important than the type of soap used. The six-step technique for hand washing is already discussed. It is also important that hands are washed under running water and not in static water, as the objective is to remove microorganisms from the hands and flush them down the drain; washing hands in static water, i.e. in a hand washbasin with a plug in, does not clean the hands as effectively as washing under running water.

ANTIBACTERIAL SOAPS   Antibacterial soaps are not required for general clinical activity; they are most useful in surgery due to their ability to lower the number of bacteria on the skin to a lower level than washing with plain soap would achieve, plus they have a residual effect, which means that it takes longer for the number of bacteria on the skin to return to normal.

Antibacterial soaps also have a cumulative effect in that the more often they are used, the greater the number of bacteria removed. Subsequently it takes longer for the number of bacteria on the skin to return to normal.

ALCOHOL HANDRUB   Alcohol handrub can be used to decontaminate the hands providing they look and feel clean. It should not be used on hands that are soiled or contaminated, as it will have no effect. Alcohol handrubs *sanitise* the hands by killing microorganisms on the skin's surface; they do not remove soil or organic matter from the skin.

- Alcohol is a disinfectant and is inactivated by dirt and organic matter. As such, if applied to a soiled or dirty hand it will not have the desired effect.
- Alcohol handrub should be applied to all surfaces of the hands and the hands rubbed until dry in order to be effective.
- The six-step technique for hand washing should be used when applying alcohol handrub.
- After 4–5 applications of alcohol handrub, hands should be washed using soap and water.
- Alcohol handrub can be used to clean the hands after removing gloves providing hands look and feel clean.
- Alcohol handrub is not reliable against the bacteria and viruses that cause diarrhoea and should not be used whenever patients have diarrhoea symptoms. Hands should be washed with soap and water at these times.
- Alcohol handrub should be applied directly to the skin – it should not be applied to gloves. Gloves should be removed and a new set donned. Gloves are single-use items and should not be cleaned and reused under any circumstances.

NAILBRUSHES   Nailbrushes should not be used as they can tear and damage the skin, creating more places for bacteria to accumulate on the hands. If used for theatre scrubbing they should be used once and discarded or returned to sterile services for decontamination before being used again.

SKIN CARE

- Any cuts or abrasions on the hands should be covered with a waterproof dressing.
- Hand cream should be applied during breaks and when off duty.

- Shared tubs or pots of hand cream should not be used, as they can become contaminated and lead to hand contamination. Pump dispensers and tubes are ideal.
- Hand creams that make it more difficult to clean the hands after application should not be used.
- Hand creams that cause any type of deterioration in glove material should not be used.

HAND ETIQUETTE   Clinical staff should have short clean nails free from dirt, nail varnish, false nails or nail attachments in order that hands can be cleaned effectively. (False nails are known to harbour more bacteria than natural nails.)

BARE BELOW THE ELBOW   It is Department of Health policy in the United Kingdom for clinical staff working with patients to be 'bare below the elbow' during clinical care activities, in order that hands can be cleaned most effectively, which is best achieved in the absence of long sleeves and hand and wrist jewellery. A plain metal band (wedding ring) can be worn but should be moved up and down the finger during hand washing in order to cleanse the skin underneath.

HAND WASHBASINS   To support effective hand washing, hand washbasins in clinical areas should have the following features:

- Mixer taps.
- Elbow/wrist/pedal/knee/sensor-operated taps, i.e. hands-free operation.
- No plug and not capable of taking a plug.
- No overflow.
- The water from the tap should not flow directly into the drainage aperture.
- Hand washbasins and taps should be wall mounted, not countersunk.

Hand washbasins in clinical areas should be used exclusively for hand washing, as using them for other activities such as emptying basins and cleaning equipment or crockery allows the sink to become contaminated, which can lead to contamination of the hands during hand washing.

Gloves, aprons, visors and masks – personal protective equipment (PPE)

This section is broken down into smaller sections on general principles of PPE use – gloves, aprons and gowns, masks, visors and goggles, headwear and footwear – and a summary of when to use PPE is included.

General principles

The principles described here apply to all situations and all clinical settings. The term PPE refers to gloves, aprons, gowns, masks, goggles and visors. The appropriate use of PPE is essential for infection control. The benefit of wearing PPE is twofold in that it provides protection to both the wearer and the patient.

Before donning PPE you should risk assess the situation – which items are most appropriate for the task/situation, depending on what you might be exposed to, e.g. blood/other body fluids? Not all items will be required each time.

You should also consider sensitivities and the risk of latex allergy (your infection control team and occupational health department will be able to advise you on local policy).

ORDER OF APPLICATION AND REMOVAL   The order of applying PPE is less critical than the order of removal – remember that when removing PPE each item is contaminated and it is important to take each item off in the correct order for your protection.

PPE should be applied in the following order:

1. Apron/gown.
2. Mask.
3. Goggles.
4. Gloves.

PPE should be removed in the following order:

1. Gloves.
2. Apron/gown.
3. Goggles.
4. Mask.

After removing PPE you must wash your hands. This is necessary to ensure that any micro-organisms that may have got on to your hands when wearing and removing PPE are not transmitted to other surfaces/patients/staff that you come into contact with.

PPE should be appropriate, fit for purpose and suitable for the person using/wearing it, with supplies located close to the point of use. It is your responsibility to ensure you have what you need, that it fits you properly and you know how to wear/use it.

PPE should be worn only when required and removed when no longer required, with hands washed immediately afterwards.

PPE should not be worn by staff when transferring patients.

Disposable gloves, aprons, gowns and masks are single-use items and their packaging will clearly state this. They should never be reused. They should be removed and disposed of when the task for which they were worn is completed, with hands washed immediately afterwards.

Reusable masks and visors must be cleaned after each use. Soapy water or a detergent wipe may be used unless blood/body fluid contamination has occurred, in which case disinfection with hypochlorite solution at 10000 parts per million available chlorine strength is required. See the section on spillage management.

Face protection should not be touched whilst being worn as this can lead to hand contamination.

Manufacturer's guidance on the use of PPE should always be adhered to.

Gloves

CHOOSING   Gloves are a medical device and should be treated as such:

- Choose the right size to ensure a good fit in order to avoid friction, excessive sweating, finger and hand muscle fatigue and interference with dexterity.
- Check the expiry date of the gloves you use – never use gloves that are out of date (glove material can deteriorate over time and an out of date glove might not perform as well).
- Never use disposable latex gloves containing powder (due to the risks associated with aerosolisation and latex allergies).

USING

- Gloves should be donned before commencing a procedure where you might come into contact with blood/body fluids/chemicals/therapeutic creams/lotions and as required for the preparation of medications.
- Gloves should be changed if they become punctured, damaged or torn, or if damage to the glove is suspected.
- Two pairs of gloves should be worn (double gloving) during some exposure prone procedures (EPPs), e.g. orthopaedic and gynaecological procedures.
- Gloves should be removed promptly after use (as soon as the procedure is complete) before touching non-contaminated/clean areas/items, environmental surfaces or other persons (including yourself), with hands washed immediately afterwards.
- Gloves being worn for a procedure/activity should not be worn to handle or write on charts, or to touch any other communal, clean surfaces.
- Gloves should not be decanted from the original box to ensure the expiry date is known and the integrity maintained.
- Gloves should never be washed or have alcohol handrub applied to them. Instead, gloves should be removed, hands cleansed and a new pair of gloves donned, if required.
- Wearing gloves does not mean that hands do not need to be washed – hands should be washed before donning gloves and after removing them.
- Jewellery should not be worn under gloves. Plain metal bands are generally tolerated but stoned rings may tear the glove material and should not be worn during clinical activity.

REMOVING   Care should be taken when removing used gloves to avoid contamination. Holding the wrist end of the glove, pull it down over itself so that it goes inside out as you pull it down your hand. Hold the removed glove in the hand that pulled it down. Now using the ungloved hand, slowly pull the other glove down, inside out, in the same way, over the fingers and the first glove and dispose of them into the clinical waste as a wrapped package.

- Gloves should be changed between patients and between procedures on the same patient to prevent cross-contamination.
- Torn, punctured or otherwise damaged gloves should not be used and should be removed immediately (safety permitting) if this occurs during a procedure.

Aprons and gowns
CHOOSING

- Aprons and gowns should be water repellent and should allow you a full range of movement when worn and not interfere with your clinical activity.
- Check expiry dates on sterile gowns before use – never use an out of date gown.

USING

- An apron or gown should be worn when contamination of your clothing or uniform might occur.
- Disposable aprons and gowns are single-use items and should be disposed of via the clinical waste stream immediately after use.
- Disposable, single-use plastic aprons should be worn when there is a risk of contact with blood/body fluids.
- An impermeable gown should be worn rather than a plastic apron when there is a risk of significant splashing of body fluids, e.g. in an operating theatre or during invasive procedures.
- Disposable long-sleeved gowns should be worn when caring for patients known or suspected to have scabies or any other parasitic skin infestation.
- Colour-coded aprons and gowns are often worn for different tasks in a ward setting, e.g. a specific colour may be worn when patients are isolated and another for serving meals – ensure that you wear the correct colour for the task in hand in accordance with local policy.
- Reusable gowns, such as those worn in operating theatres, should be worn once and then laundered. They must be changed between patients.
- Disposable aprons and gowns must never be cleaned and reused.
- An apron or gown should be worn for one patient and then removed. It may be necessary to change your apron or gown between tasks on the same patient to prevent cross-contamination.
- A torn or damaged apron or gown should not be used and should be removed immediately (safety permitting) if this occurs during a procedure.
- An apron or gown should be removed as soon as the task for which it was worn is complete, before touching non-contaminated and clean areas, items, environmental surfaces and contact with other patients and staff.

REMOVING

- When removing an apron or gown you should avoid touching the most heavily soiled/contaminated areas. You should also take care not to touch your clothing or uniform worn underneath to avoid contamination.
- Turn the outer contaminated side of the gown inward, roll the aprons or gown into a ball and dispose of it via the clinical waste stream.

Masks
CHOOSING

- A wide range of masks are available: reusable and disposable surgical and FFP3 masks; masks with visors; masks without visors, etc. Make sure you know what is available in your place of work, how to wear it and how to use it – always follow the manufacturer's guidance on use, make sure each item fits comfortably and check expiry dates.
- If there is any possibility that blood, body fluids, medications or fluids of any type may be splashed in your face, you should wear a surgical mask.

- If you are caring for someone with an infection that is transmitted via the airborne route, e.g. influenza, and will be performing an aerosol generating procedure such as intubation, oro/nasopharyngeal suctioning, tracheostomy care, chest physiotherapy, bronchoscopy/CPR, etc., you should wear an FFP3 mask.
- Manufacturers' instructions should be adhered to while donning masks to ensure the most appropriate fit and optimum protection.

USING   The purpose of wearing a mask is to prevent splashes from going in your mouth or up your nose. Specialist masks also filter the air you breathe. Torn or damaged masks should not be worn as they may not provide the desired level of protection.

SURGICAL MASKS   These provide a physical barrier against splashes to the mouth and nose. They do not filter the air you inhale and are not an effective barrier for fine aerosol droplets that float through the air and are inhaled. Care should be taken to ensure that surgical masks fit snugly around the nose and chin.

Surgical masks are single-use, disposable items and should be removed when no longer required. They should not be worn around the neck and should be changed when moist/wet/contaminated.

FILTERING FACEPIECE MASKS (FFP MASKS)   These provide a physical barrier against splashes to the mouth and nose and also filter the air you inhale. They are capable of filtering fine aerosols. FFP3 masks are the mask of choice, providing a higher level of filtration than FFP2 masks.

FFP3 masks should be worn when aerosolising procedures are underway with patients with infections transmitted via the airborne route, e.g. influenza, tuberculosis, etc. They must be fitted to ensure the best possible fit on to your face. A 'fit test' should be carried out to check how well the mask fits (Box 1).

Box 1   Fit test for masks

FFP3 mask fit testing

- Fit testing is a one-off test but should be repeated if facial shape changes/following significant weight gain/loss.
- FFP3 fit testing is a legal requirement.
- The wearer must achieve an adequate fit with each specific model of FFP3.

Factors affecting face seal

- Jewellery – may need to be removed.
- Facial markings, e.g. scar/mole.
- Safety or prescription glasses (should be worn during fit test).
- Facial hair. A small goatee or beard than will be covered by the mask may be okay, otherwise staff must be clean shaven for a proper fit and face seal. Otherwise, those with facial hair should shave/do not perform aerosolising procedures/use a hood with powered extraction.

Carry out a fit check before the fit test

- Cover the mask surface with flat hands. For valved masks inhale sharply and for unvalved masks exhale sharply. If leaks around the seal are detected, correctly fit the mask before entering a hazardous area.

REMOVING   When removing disposable masks the outer contaminated side of the mask should be turned inward upon removal and the masks disposed of via the clinical waste stream.

Visors and goggles (eye protection), headwear and footwear

CHOOSING   Goggles should protect you against splashes to your eyes. They should wrap around the eye area to ensure side areas are protected.

Visors may be worn instead of a mask and goggle combination when there is a high risk of splattering or spray of blood or other body fluids.

USING

- Visors/goggles should be worn to protect the eyes whenever there is a risk of splashing to the face. They should be removed when no longer required.
- Visors/goggles should be worn during aerosol generating procedures (intubation, oro/nasopharyngeal suctioning, tracheostomy care, chest physiotherapy, bronchoscopy/cardiopulmonary resuscitation).
- Visors/goggles should be worn by all theatre staff directly participating in an invasive procedure where there is a risk of splashing to the face.
- Torn or otherwise damaged face protection should not be used and should be removed immediately (safety permitting) if this occurs during a procedure.

REMOVING   Remove goggles/visors promptly after use, avoiding contact with most likely contaminated areas, e.g. the front surface. This should be done by handling the straps/ear loops/goggle legs only (manufacturers' instructions should be followed).

HEADWARE   Theatre hats should be worn in theatres, sterile services departments and clean rooms. They should cover the hair entirely and should be changed between sessions or if contaminated with blood or body fluids.

FOOTWARE   Footwear should be clean and well maintained. It should support and cover the whole foot to protect from dropped sharps and blood/body fluid spillages. Footwear dedicated to a specific clinical area, such as theatre, should be removed before leaving that area.

Summary of when to use PPE

The guidance contained within Table 1 is not exhaustive; it offers examples of common care activities where blood/other body fluid exposure may occur and protection must be worn. As standard, a risk assessment must be undertaken to consider the risks of blood/other body fluid exposure prior to activities. For further information refer to your local infection control team/policy.

Table 1 Summary of when to use PPE

Activity	Aprons/gowns (depending on significant splashing/ exposure)	Face, eye, mouth protection (surgical masks, goggles)	Gloves
Contact with intact skin – no visible blood/ body fluids, rashes	Not required	Not required	Not required
Sterile procedures	Required	Risk assessment	Required
Contact with wounds, skin lesions	Required	Risk assessment	Required
Managing spillages of urine and faeces	Required	Risk assessment	Required
Potential exposure to blood/other body fluids, e.g. performing suctioning, cleaning up spillages, taking specimens	Required	Risk assessment	Required
Venepuncture/cannulation	Required	Not required	Required
Vaginal examination	Required	Not required	Required
Applying topical creams, etc.	Not required	Not required	Required
Touching patients with unknown skin rash	Risk assessment	Not required	Required
Emptyichanging urinary catheter bags, urinals, bedpans, etc.	Required	Risk assessment	Required
Handling specimens	Required	Not required	Required
Handling used instruments	Required	Not required	Required
Using disinfectants, cleaning agents	Required	Risk assessment	Required
General cleaning of clinical areas and equipment	Risk assessment	Not required	Risk assessment
Bed making, dressing patients	Risk assessment	Not required	Risk assessment
Oral care	Risk assessment	Risk assessment	Required
Feeding patient	Required	Not required	Risk assessment
Handling waste	Risk assessment	Risk assessment	Required

Decontamination

This section is broken down into several sections and includes cleaning and disinfection of healthcare equipment and the healthcare environment.

Definitions and application of processes

The term 'decontamination' refers to the combination of processes by which pathogenic microorganisms, including bacterial spores, are removed from an item, making it safe to handle, use or discard. Decontamination is a three-step process that involves cleaning, disinfection and sterilisation (in that order).

CLEANING   Cleaning is a process that uses detergent and water to remove visible contamination. It does not necessarily destroy microbes. Effective cleaning is essential before disinfection or sterilisation. It is imperative that detergent is used to clean, not disinfectant.

Detergent is crucial in cleaning as it breaks up dirt and grease, making it easier for the water to remove any contamination. The combination of detergent and water removes around 80% of microorganisms from surfaces.

Drying after cleaning is as important as cleaning itself in order to prevent growth of microorganisms not removed during the cleaning process; this is true for hands and surfaces.

DISINFECTION   Disinfection is a process that uses chemical agents or heat to eliminate many or all pathogenic microorganisms on inanimate objects, with the exception of bacterial spores.

Disinfectants should only be used when there is a risk of transmission of infection, e.g. when a patient has an infection. They are not required routinely; cleaning with detergent alone is adequate.

Disinfectants should be used to disinfect. They should be applied to clean surfaces – they must not be used to clean (with the exception of products used for blood/body fluid spillage management).

Alcohol is a disinfectant (not a cleanser) and should not be used for cleaning. Alcohol acts as a fixative to proteins (which are present in blood and tissue) and makes them stick to surfaces.

STERILISATION   This is the complete elimination or destruction of all forms of microbial life, including bacterial spores.

INFECTION RISKS AND DECONTAMINATION REQUIREMENTS   It is important when buying equipment to check with the manufacturer how it should be decontaminated and that the recommended method is achievable, as to deviate from manufacturer's guidance may invalidate the product warranty and transfer liability for the product (should it fail or cause harm) to you as the user.

Decontamination of reusable medical devices should be undertaken in a dedicated facility that ensures segregation of dirty and clean items, has a defined workflow, moving from dirty to clean, and supports tracking and tracing of individual items, with documentation that supports this, e.g. a sterile services department (SSD). Local decontamination at ward level should be avoided.

The level of decontamination an item requires is dependent on how it is used – non-invasive items require a lower level of decontamination than invasive items (see Table 2).

Table 2 Infection risks and decontamination requirements

Level of risk	Application	Level of decontamination required	Examples
High	Invasive items Items in close contact with a break in the skin or mucous membrane Items introduced into a sterile body area	Sterilisation High-level disinfection may be adequate for some items	Surgical instruments Dressings Catheters Prosthetic devices
Intermediate	Items in contact with intact mucous membranes, body fluids Items contaminated with particularly virulent or readily transmissible organisms Items for use on highly susceptible patients or sites	Disinfection	Endoscopes Respiratory equipment
Low	Items in contact with normal/intact skin	Cleaning and drying Disinfection is required if there is a known risk of infection	Washbowls Toilets Bedding
Minimal	Items not in contact with the patient/their immediate surroundings	Cleaning and drying	Floors Sinks Walls

SINGLE USE ONLY   Items designated 'single use only' by the manufacturer must not be reused under any circumstances, despite any cost concerns. Figure 2 shows the 'single use only' symbol.

DO NOT REUSE

Figure 2   Single use only symbol

When the 'single use only' symbol is seen on a medical device or its packaging the item must be used once only and discarded. This is different from single-patient use items that can be reused with the same patient.

If single-use items are reprocessed (decontaminated) and reused, the product liability is transferred from the manufacturer to the reprocessor, who becomes responsible for the item's performance. This means that if a product fails to operate properly or causes harm or injury it is the responsibility of the reprocessor.

Decontamination of healthcare equipment

- All items of equipment should be cleaned after each use/between patients.
- Manufacturer's guidance must be adhered to when cleaning healthcare equipment.

Table 3   Healthcare equipment and decontamination methods

Item	Decontamination method – all items require decontamination after each use
Beds	Wash bed frame with detergent and water If disinfection is required use a chlorine-releasing agent at 1000 parts per million available chlorine strength
Bed cradles	Wash with detergent and water If disinfection is required use a chlorine-releasing agent at 1000 parts per million available chlorine strength
Commode frame	Clean with detergent wipes If disinfection is required use a chlorine-releasing agent at 1000 parts per million available chlorine strength Commodes should be disassembled for cleaning and disinfection
Commode pan	Wash with detergent and water If disinfection is required use a chlorine-releasing agent at 1000 parts per million available chlorine strength
Reusable bedpans	Wash in an automated washer–disinfector with a heat disinfection cycle that reaches 90 °C, or reaches 80 °C and maintains the temperature for 1 minute OR Wash in detergent and water then disinfect with a chlorine-releasing agent at 1000 parts per million available chlorine strength
Bedpan holder (used with disposable liners)	Wash with detergent and water If disinfection is required use a chlorine-releasing agent at 1000 parts per million available chlorine strength
Blood pressure cuffs	Wipe with a detergent wipe If disinfection is required use a chlorine-releasing agent at 1000 parts per million available chlorine strength
Dressings trolleys	Wash with detergent and water To disinfect wipe with 70% alcohol after cleaning
Incubator	Wash with detergent and water If disinfection is required use a chlorine-releasing agent at 125 parts per million available chlorine strength or wipe surfaces with 70% alcohol
Mattresses	Wash with detergent and water avoiding excess wetting If disinfection is required use a chlorine-releasing agent at 1000 parts per million available chlorine strength
Nailbrushes	Sterilised by heat disinfection in SSD
Pillows	Wash with detergent and water avoiding excess wetting If disinfection is required use a chlorine-releasing agent at 1000 parts per million available chlorine strength
Portable suction unit	Wash bottle in detergent and water after emptying, after each use If contents were blood stained, disinfect after washing with a chlorine-releasing agent at 10000 parts per million available chlorine
Sheets	Send for laundering at patient discharge/when soiled/stained/contaminated/creased, at least twice a week
Thermometers	After removal of protective sleeve disinfect with an alcohol wipe
Toys	Wash hard toys with detergent and water If disinfection is required use a chlorine-releasing agent at 1000 parts per million available chlorine strength and rinse or wipe with 70% alcohol
Urine bottles	Wash in an automated washer–disinfector with a heat disinfection cycle that reaches 90 °C, or reaches 80 °C and maintains the temperature for 1 minute OR Wash in detergent and water and then disinfect with a chlorine-releasing agent at 1000 parts per million available chlorine strength
Wash bowls (plastic)	Wash with detergent and water and dry thoroughly

- General purpose detergent and water/detergent wipes should be suitable for cleaning the majority of items. Consult your infection control team and decontamination manager for further advice and always follow manufacturer's guidance when cleaning equipment in order to avoid causing damage.
- Wear an apron and gloves when cleaning.

Table 3 sets out the cleaning and disinfection methods for items of healthcare equipment commonly used at ward level. This guidance may differ from local policy – please refer to infection control guidance in your place of work.

Note that disinfection is required if an item was used with an infectious patient. If contamination with high-risk blood or body fluid occurs, a chlorine-releasing agent at 10000 parts per million available chlorine strength should be used to disinfect. Check manufacturer's guidance beforehand for compatibility and refer to the subsection on management of blood and body fluid spillages and splashes.

Decontamination of the healthcare environment

GENERAL STANDARDS

- All areas must be kept free of unnecessary equipment and clutter to facilitate cleaning.
- The healthcare environment and all patient equipment must be visibly clean and free from dust, dirt, debris and blood/body fluid contamination/ stains.
- The floor should not be used for storage – floors must be kept clear to facilitate cleaning.
- The fabric of the environment should be maintained and any damage or defects should be repaired/replaced.
- Every bed space/single room should be cleaned with detergent and water when a patient leaves before the next patient is admitted.
- Cleaning schedules should be displayed publicly.

ISOLATION ROOMS

- Isolation rooms should be cleaned last after all other areas in the ward to prevent the spread of microorganisms and transmission of infection.
- The domestic should wear disposable gloves and an apron when cleaning in an isolation room. These should be removed in the room immediately before leaving, discarded into the clinical waste bag and hands should be washed.
- On a daily basis the room should be cleaned with detergent and water and then disinfected using a chlorine-releasing agent at 1000 parts per million available chlorine strength or cleaned and disinfected in one step with a chlorine-based detergent at 1000 parts per million available chlorine strength.
- After discharge of an infectious patient the room should be cleaned with detergent and water and then disinfected using a chlorine-releasing agent at 1000 parts per million available chlorine strength or cleaned and disinfected in one step with a chlorine-based detergent at 1000 parts per million available chlorine strength.
- Curtains should be changed after the patient is discharged/transferred from the ward.

CURTAINS

- Curtains should be changed when soiled/contaminated, after outbreaks of infection, after discharge of an isolated patient and otherwise every three months as a minimum.
- Fabric curtains should be laundered every three months and disposable curtains should be changed every three months as a matter of routine.

- If curtains become stained, contaminated or soiled they must be changed immediately.
- No curtain should be stained – curtains with old stains that are set into the fabric should not be used.

EQUIPMENT USED FOR CLEANING

- The domestic should wear heavy-duty gloves for cleaning, not disposable clinical gloves, unless working in an isolation room.
- Mops and buckets should be stored clean, dry and upside down to allow drying and to avoid dust and debris from accumulating inside. Buckets should be stacked in a pyramid style, not inside one another.
- Cleaning materials used by the ward domestic should be stored in the domestic service room and not in any other area of the ward.
- Cloths used to clean and disinfect isolation rooms should be disposable or laundered immediately after cleaning the isolation room. They must not be used to clean another area.
- All mop heads and cloths should be laundered daily.

COLOUR CODING FOR HYGIENE   The following colour-coding scheme should be applied to all cleaning materials (gloves, mop handles, buckets, cloths):

Red: bathrooms, washrooms, showers, toilets, basins and bathroom floors
Blue: general areas including wards, departments, offices and basins in public areas
Green: catering departments, ward kitchen areas and patient food service at ward level
Yellow: isolation areas

DOMESTIC SERVICE ROOM (CLEANER'S CUPBOARD)   The domestic service room should be used solely to prepare and clean equipment used for cleaning; there should be no personal belongings stored and food should not be consumed there. The domestic service room is regarded as a dirty environment in the same way that the sluice room is, and to consume food there presents a risk of infection to the member of staff.

CLEANING FREQUENCIES
Blinds and curtains
In a hospital setting, curtains and blinds should be changed every three months and immediately upon soiling, staining or contamination.

Floors
Floors should be washed daily with detergent and water. Spillages should be cleaned (and disinfected if necessary) immediately.

Horizontal surfaces
All horizontal surfaces should be cleaned daily with detergent and water.

Lockers, bed tables
Lockers and bed tables should be washed daily with detergent and water. Spillages should be cleaned (and disinfected if necessary) immediately.

Showers
Shower curtains should be cleaned daily with detergent and water and changed every three months – sooner if contaminated.

Toilets
Toilets should be cleaned daily as a minimum and more frequently during outbreaks of diarrhoeal illness, when they should be disinfected with a chlorine-releasing agent at 1000

parts per million available chlorine strength. Toilets should be cleaned at any time that they are soiled.

Walls
In theatres walls should be cleaned every 6 months. In other areas there is no requirement to wash walls with any specified frequency other than to spot-clean any areas that become dirty using detergent and water.

Wash hand basins
Wash hand basins should be cleaned daily as a minimum and more frequently during out-breaks of diarrhoeal illness, when they should be disinfected with a chlorine-releasing agent at 1000 parts per million available chlorine strength.

Windows
Window cleaning is usually done by an external contractor and there is no recommended frequency.

Managing blood and body fluid spillages and splashes
Blood and body fluids have different levels of risk in terms of their infectivity – see the subsection on infectivity of body fluids.

In the event of a blood/body fluid spillage it is essential to disinfect the affected area as described here in order to avoid transmission of bloodborne viruses. Hepatitis B can survive on surfaces for at least seven days and it is possible to pick it up from inanimate objects; therefore careful disinfection of spillages and contamination is essential.

HAND HYGIENE, GLOVES, APRONS, VISORS AND MASKS

- When disinfecting spillages gloves and an apron should be worn.
- If there is any risk of splashing to the face a surgical mask and eye protection should also be worn.
- After dealing with the spillage the gloves, apron, etc., should be removed and hands should be washed.

DISINFECTING THE SPILLAGE   Hypochlorite preparations should be used to disinfect spillages, at the following concentrations:

- 1000 parts per million available chlorine for urine, vomit or faeces.
- 10000 parts per million available chlorine for blood/body fluid spillages.
- If hypochlorite solution at 10000 parts per million available chlorine has already been prepared and the weaker solution has not, it is acceptable to use the stronger solution to disinfect following spillage of urine, vomit or faeces – preparation of a separate solution is not strictly necessary.

Hypochlorite granules should be used for fresh blood/body fluid spillages; these absorb the spillage whilst disinfecting with 10000 parts per million available chlorine.

- Do not apply hypochlorite granules to urine or vomit spillages, as the chemical reaction that occurs causes chlorine gas to be released.

A wide range of products are available for managing blood and body fluid spill-ages, including biohazard kits, impregnated wipes – make sure you are familiar with the products available in your organisation and how to use them.

BLOOD/BLOOD-STAINED BODY FLUIDS

Fresh spillages

1. Apply hypochlorite granules to the affected area and leave for two minutes.
2. Clear up the spillage and granules with paper products, i.e. disposable items, and discard into clinical waste.
3. Wash the affected area using general purpose detergent and water or detergent wipes to remove residual hypochlorite.
4. Dry the affected area thoroughly.

Dried blood/blood-stained body fluids/splashes/ environmental contamination

1. Apply hypochlorite solution at 10000 parts per million available chlorine strength to the affected area using paper products. Allow two minutes contact time for disinfection to take place. Where this is not practicable, e.g. splashes on equipment, hypochlorite solution should be used to wipe the equipment to remove the contamination.
2. Discard all paper products used to clear up the spillage into a clinical waste bag.
3. Wash the affected area using general purpose detergent and water or detergent wipes to remove residual hypochlorite.
4. Dry the affected area thoroughly.

URINE, VOMIT AND FAECES

1. Clear up the urine/vomit/faeces with paper products and discard into a clinical waste bag.
2. Disinfect the affected area using paper products and hypochlorite solution at 1000 parts per million available chlorine strength.
3. Wash the affected area using detergent and water or detergent wipes to remove residual hypochlorite and then dry thoroughly.
4. A chlorine-based detergent at 1000 parts per million available chlorine strength can be used instead of steps 2 and 3.

INFECTIVITY OF BODY FLUIDS   Body fluids are regarded as being 'high risk' or 'low risk' in terms of infectivity. Urine, vomit and faeces are low risk; the following are high risk:

• Blood/blood-stained body fluids
• Semen
• Vaginal secretions
• Synovial fluid
• Cerebrospinal fluid
• Amniotic fluid (liquor)
• Peritoneal fluid
• Pleural fluid
• Breast milk.

CARE WITH HYPOCHLORITE PREPARATIONS

• Always prepare hypochlorite solution(s) in the container(s) provided by the manufacturer. There should be two available to you – one for 10000 parts per million available chlorine concentration and another for 1000 parts per million available chlorine concentration.
• Follow manufacturer's guidance on preparation of the solution(s).
• Prepare with cold water.

- Do not decant the solution into another vessel.
- Do not shake the container whilst waiting for the tablets to dissolve as to do so may lead to the contents spraying out when the lid is removed.
- Hypochlorite solutions lose their strength after 24 hours – discard any unused solution(s) after 24 hours and prepare a fresh batch the next time it is needed.
- Keep the lid of the container – the container should not be used without a lid.
- Hypochlorite solutions are COSHH substances and should be stored securely.
- Hypochlorite is corrosive to metal and therefore prolonged contact with metal should be avoided.
- Manufacturer's guidance should be consulted before applying hypochlorite solution to any item of equipment.
- Do not apply hypochlorite to carpets and soft furnishings as it will strip out the colour; instead clean with general purpose detergent and water and use steam to disinfect.
- Heavily soiled/contaminated items that cannot be cleaned and disinfected must be discarded.
- The products used to clear up spillages must all be disposable – mops and buckets should not be used.

Isolation and cohorting

Isolation and cohorting are sometimes required to prevent the transmission of infection. This section is broken down into smaller sections that discuss use of isolation facilities, isolation precautions and cohorting. A summary of the infections that necessitate isolation is included.

Use of isolation facilities

RISK ASSESSMENT   When admitting a patient known or suspected to have an infection the following should be considered when deciding what type of ward to admit them to and whether they require an isolation room:

- How dangerous is the infection? Is it life threatening or capable of causing severe disease?
- How easily can the infection be transmitted – what is the route of transmission?
- What is best for the patient?
- What is the best way to manage the risk of infection to other patients and staff?
- Susceptibility of other patients in the ward.
- What would the impact be (if any) on the organisation if there were an outbreak of this infection, in terms of continuation of services, reputation?
- Availability of an isolation room.

REQUIREMENT FOR ISOLATION   Patients known or suspected to have an infection should be nursed in isolation to prevent the spread of infection to others. Guidance on isolation room priority follows, but, as a general rule, patients with pyrexia of unknown origin, an unexplained rash or diarrhoea (with or without vomiting) should be isolated as a precautionary measure until a possible infectious cause has been ruled out. Patients with suspected infectious diarrhoea should be isolated promptly due to the highly infectious nature of diarrhoeal illnesses such as norovirus. Isolation of infectious patients is sometimes referred to as 'source' or 'standard' isolation or 'barrier nursing'.

Patients who are particularly vulnerable to infection should be isolated to minimise their risk of becoming infected, e.g. neutropenic patients. This is sometimes referred to as 'protective' isolation or 'reverse barrier nursing'.

Patients with rare, highly infectious diseases, such as Ebola virus, should be isolated. This is sometimes referred to as 'strict' isolation and usually takes place in a designated infectious diseases hospital and as such is not discussed further here.

ALLOCATION OF ISOLATION ROOMS   At times the availability of single rooms to isolate patients may be limited and the demand for isolation rooms may exceed availability. Patients who are infectious have a higher priority for single rooms than disruptive patients and those nearing the end of life, which is often a contentious issue and somewhat controversial. The importance of protecting patients from infection must be given priority.

Some infections are more easily transmittable than others and more serious in terms of the problems they cause. Where isolation room availability is limited a risk assessment is required in order to prioritise isolation room allocation. It is essential to discuss isolation and cohorting with the local infection control and bed management teams before considering moving patients.

The risk of transmission of infection is increased when bed occupancy rates are high, there is increased movement of patients between wards and departments, and when the demand for isolation rooms exceeds availability.

Allocation of isolation rooms should be based upon a risk assessment in order to make the best use of existing facilities. Where the need for isolation rooms exceeds availability it may be necessary to nurse patients with the same infection together in one area, which is known as cohorting. Decisions on isolation and cohorting should be made in consultation with bed managers and infection control teams.

NEGATIVE PRESSURE ROOMS   Patients with infectious conditions that are transmitted via the airborne route should be nursed in a negative pressure room wherever possible. This includes multidrug-resistant tuberculosis (MDR-TB), measles and chickenpox. In a negative pressure room the direction of airflow is from the corridor into the room and out through an extract, which prevents contaminated air and droplets from being blown out of the room into the corridor and ward environment.

Whilst negative pressure rooms are beneficial they are not essential. Prevention of transmission of airborne infections can be achieved without negative pressure ventilation through strict adherence to the guidance given here.

Isolation precautions

Isolation precautions are essentially the same for protective and source isolation. With source isolation the object is to avoid bringing microorgansms out of the isolation environment and transferring them to others. In protective isolation the object is to avoid taking microorganisms from the ward into the environment of a particularly vulnerable patient. When caring for a patient in isolation the following precautions are required.

PATIENT MANAGEMENT, PLACEMENT AND MOVEMENT

- The patient must be informed of the requirement to nurse them in isolation and the rationale for doing so. They should be advised of what being nursed in isolation entails, e.g. that they should not leave the room. It is important that the isolation requirements are explained to the patient and their visitors in order to alleviate their anxiety and increase the likelihood of compliance.
- The patient should be nursed in a single room, preferably with an en suite toilet.
- Their movement in and out of the room must be restricted.
- Isolated patients cannot leave their rooms for occupational therapy and physiotherapy.
- Movement of an isolated patient to other departments for investigations must be risk assessed, based upon the seriousness of their condition and the urgency of the investigation compared with the risk of transmission of infection to others/exposure of the vulnerable patient to microorganisms. If not urgent, the investigation should be delayed.
- If an infectious patient is moved to another ward/department the receiving area must be informed of the patient's infectious status in order that they can take the relevant infection control precautions.
- Wounds must be covered and if the patient has an infection transmitted via the airborne/droplet route they should wear a mask for the duration of the time that they are out of the isolation room.
- Ideally the infectious patient should be seen last on a list or as late in the day as possible.
- The infectious patient must not be kept waiting in a communal area.
- All equipment used with an infectious patient must be cleaned after use.
- The environment must be cleaned and disinfected before other patients are treated there, using a chlorine-releasing agent at 1000 parts per million available chlorine strength or 10000 parts per million available chlorine strength if blood spillage/contamination occurs.
- Porters should wear gloves and aprons when assisting the patient from their bed/chair on to a wheelchair/trolley and remove them and wash their hands before taking the patient out of the isolation room.

GLOVES, APRONS, VISORS AND MASKS

- Gloves and aprons (and masks and visors if required) should be available outside the room.
- Ideally, gloves, aprons, masks and visors should not be stored inside isolation rooms as they can become contaminated. If they are available inside the room they should be discarded when the patient is discharged.
- All staff caring for the patient should wear gloves and an apron for patient contact.
- A clinical waste bin must be available in the room for disposal of gloves and aprons.
- Gloves and aprons must be removed prior to leaving the room and hands washed.

INFORMATION FOR STAFF AND VISITORS

- An isolation sign should be placed on the door to alert everyone that isolation precautions are in place.
- The isolation sign should indicate if masks and goggles/visors are required.
- The reason for isolating the patient must be documented in the notes.
- There should be a review date recorded in the notes or on the isolation sign.

MAINTAINING ISOLATION PRECAUTIONS

- Doors to isolation rooms must remain closed unless the patient requires observation.
- If it is not safe to maintain isolation precautions for any reason this must be documented in the notes, e.g. a patient at risk of falling.
- The number of staff entering the room must be restricted to a minimum to protect staff from the risk of infection and to reduce the risk of staff transmitting the infection to other patients.
- Therapists should ideally see all other patients on the ward before the infected isolated patient or see the isolated vulnerable patient first.

EQUIPMENT

- Observation charts and notes should be stored outside the room to reduce the need to enter the isolation environment.
- It is especially important that equipment is cleaned before being taking into the isolation room of a vulnerable patient and after use with an infectious patient.
- Ideally, equipment used with a patient in isolation should remain in the isolation room with them and not be used with anyone else until isolation precautions are no longer required.
- Equipment and furniture in the isolation room must be restricted to that which is essential to minimise the risk of contamination.
- Fans should not be used where patients with infections spread by droplet or aerosol transmission are being cared for.
- Patients in isolation can use the same crockery and cutlery as other patients.

LINEN AND LAUNDRY

- All used linen and laundry should be treated as 'infected' and placed in a red bag. When the bag becomes full it must be removed from the isolation room and taken to the used linen storage facility.
- Extra items of clean linen should not be stored in an isolation room as it may become contaminated. Any unused linen items stored in an isolation room must be sent for laundering; they must not be returned to the linen store.

CLEANING AND DISINFECTION

- Isolation rooms should be cleaned and disinfected daily and after patient discharge with detergent followed by a chlorine-releasing agent at 1000 parts per million available chlorine strength or cleaned and disinfected in one step using a chlorine-based detergent at 1000 parts per million available chlorine strength.
- After discharge the curtains should be changed.
- Cloths and mops used in isolation rooms must be laundered immediately after use and not use anywhere else on the ward.
- When an isolation room is vacated it must be thoroughly cleaned and disinfected before another patient is placed there.

VISITORS

- Visiting should be restricted and it is generally advisable to exclude children.
- Visitors with cold or flu symptoms should wait until their symptoms have completely gone before visiting.
- Visitors with diarrhoea and vomiting must not visit until they have been symptom-free for 48 hours.
- Information leaflets should be available for visitors on some common infectious conditions such as norovirus, MRSA and *Clostridium difficile*.
- Visitors need not wear gloves and aprons whilst visiting unless they provide care for the patient. If they choose to wear gloves and aprons they must be informed that the gloves and apron must be removed in the room and hands washed before leaving and the reason why this is important.
- Visitors should always wash their hands before leaving an isolation room/bay.

Cohorting

When nursing patients with the same infection in a cohort the isolation precautions described above should be applied, with the following additions:

- Gloves and aprons worn in a cohort area/bay should be changed between patients and hands washed – it is not acceptable to wear a pair of gloves and an apron to enter the area and to keep them on whilst moving from patient to patient as this can lead to transmission of infection.
- Equipment in the cohort area/bay must be cleaned in between patients.
- Notes trolleys should not be taken into an area where a group of infectious patients are being cared for.
- A patient with diarrhoea being nursed in a cohort area who is unable to mobilise to the toilet should be provided with a commode specifically for his or her individual use that is not shared with anyone else. The commode must be cleaned and disinfected after each use.
- When taking bedpans, urinals, commodes, etc., to the dirty utility room for disposal it is acceptable to wear the gloves and apron worn in the isolation room providing they are removed immediately afterwards and hands are washed.

Isolation priority and duration

Table 4 lists a range of conditions, their priority for isolation facilities and the length of time that isolation is required.

Table 4   Isolation priority and duration

Infection/condition/ circumstance	Isolation room required	Stop isolation
Acinetobacter (multiresistant)	Essential	Maintain isolation indefinitely Seek advice from the infection control team
Admitted from another hospital/care home	Preferred	If MRSA screening swabs are negative and there are no signs of infection
Campylobacter	Essential	48 hours after symptoms have resolved
Chickenpox	Essential	When all spots have crusted over
Clostridium difficile	Essential	When patient has type 3 or 4 stools
Diarrhoea	Essential	48 hours after symptoms have resolved
Enterobacter (multiresistant)	Essential if present in sputum and patient coughing	Maintain isolation indefinitely Seek advice from the infection control team
ESBL	Essential in ITU Preferable in other areas	Maintain isolation indefinitely Seek advice from the infection control team
Group A *Streptococcus*	Essential	• 24 hours after treatment commenced • When swab results are negative
Hepatitis A	Preferred	After the first week of jaundice
Hepatitis B	Not required unless the patient is bleeding	
Hepatitis C	Not required unless the patient is bleeding	
HIV	Not required	
Influenza	Essential	When symptoms have resolved
Klebsiella (multiresistant)	Essential if present in sputum and patient coughing	Maintain isolation indefinitely Seek advice from the infection control team
Legionella	Not required	
Lice (head, body and pubic)	Not required	
Measles	Essential	Four days after rash first appeared
Meningitis (bacterial)	Essential	24 hours after treatment commenced
Meningitis (viral)	Preferred	When symptoms have resolved
MRSA	Essential in orthopaedics, surgery, oncology and haematology Preferred in medical wards, particularly if present in sputum and patient coughing, or patient has an exfoliative skin condition such as eczema	After three sets of negative screening swabs
Mumps	Essential	Five days after onset of symptoms
Neutropenia	Essential for patients post bone marrow transplant/ chemotherapy	When white cell count is normal
Norovirus	Essential	48 hours after symptoms have resolved
Patients receiving palliative/end of life care	Preferred	If isolation room is required for an infectious patient
Patients who are disruptive	Preferred	If isolation room is required for an infectious patient
Pneumococcus (penicillin resistant)	Preferred	Maintain isolation indefinitely Seek advice from the infection control team

Table 4 Continued

Infection/condition/ circumstance	Isolation room required	Stop isolation
Pyrexia of unknown origin	Essential	• Until infection is ruled out • If an infectious cause is identified the isolation precautions for that condition must be applied
Rash	Essential	
Respiratory syncytial virus (RSV)	Preferred	When symptoms have resolved
Rotavirus	Essential	48 hours after symptoms have resolved
Rubella	Essential	4 days after onset of rash
Scabies (classical)	Essential	12–24 hours after **first** treatment was applied (depending on preparation used)
Scabies (crusted)	Essential	12–24 hours after **final** treatment applied (depending on preparation used)
Shingles	Essential	When all lesions have crusted over
Stenotrophomonas	Preferred in intensive care and high-dependency units	Maintain isolation indefinitely Seek advice from the infection control team
Tuberculosis (pulmonary), includes multidrug-resistant tuberculosis (MDR-TB)	Essential Negative pressure room preferred for MDR-TB	Two weeks after treatment commenced
Vancomycin-resistant *Enterococci* (VRE)	Essential	Never – maintain isolation throughout hospital stay and at every admission
Viral haemorrhagic fever	Essential, preferably in a specialist infectious diseases unit	Maintain isolation for the duration of admission
Whooping cough	Essential	Three weeks after onset of symptoms

Respiratory precautions, respiratory hygiene and cough etiquette

Depending on the type of organism, surfaces involved and level of contamination, the pathogens that cause respiratory tract infections can survive in the environment for a limited period of time. Influenza can be picked up via the hands from contaminated hard surfaces for up to 24 hours after contamination occurred and from contaminated soft surfaces such as clothing, tissues and magazines for up to two hours; therefore respiratory precautions are essential. Respiratory tract infections are spread by the following routes:

1. Droplet transmission. Large droplets (generated during coughing, sneezing and talking) from an infected person can cause infection in another person if mucous membrane contact occurs by entering the mouth or nose or coming into contact with the surface of the eye. These large droplets are too heavy to remain suspended in the air and land within a metre of the patient; therefore those coming within one metre of the infectious patient are at risk of infection.
2. Airborne droplet transmission (in aerosol generating procedures). Aerosol generating procedures can make a very fine mist of the patient's secretions, with droplets small and light enough to float through the air. These small droplets can travel for over a metre; therefore those not in direct contact with the patient are also at risk of infection. Transmission of infection can occur if the droplets are inhaled or if mucous membrane contact occurs by entry of the droplets to the mouth or nose, or if they come into contact with the surface of the eye.
3. Direct contact transmission. When an infected person coughs/sneezes on to their hands and then touches another person, transmission of infection can occur when the other person touches their mouth, nose or eyes.
4. Indirect contact transmission. Any item (equipment, bedding, furniture) used by or with an infected person is contaminated and if reused can lead to transmission of infection. Microorganisms present on the used item can be transferred by the next user to their eyes, nose and mouth and cause infection.

Preventing transmission of infection

The standard principles of infection control should be applied at all times by all staff, even if they have had the infection previously or have been vaccinated against it.

PATIENT PLACEMENT

- Isolate the patient (single room priority should be given to patients who are coughing and producing sputum excessively, as they pose the greatest risk of transmission of infection to others).
- If a single room is not available, the patient should be cohorted with patients who have the same infection. Beds should be more than one metre apart and curtains between beds should be drawn to minimise the risk of patients having close contact with one another.
- Isolation signs should be used on isolation rooms/cohort bays.
- Movement of the patient out of the single room/cohort bay should be avoided unless medically urgent. If transfer is essential the patient should wear a surgical mask to contain their secretions.
- Isolation precautions should be maintained for 24 hours after the patient's fever and respiratory symptoms have resolved.
- In prolonged illness with complications such as pneumonia, isolation precautions should be maintained until the patient has improved clinically.

- Those who are immunosuppressed or seriously ill can remain infectious for longer than those who are immunocompetent. The decision to discontinue isolation precautions in these patients must be based upon their clinical condition and in agreement with the local infection control team.

PERSONAL PROTECTIVE EQUIPMENT

- A surgical facemask should be worn when working in close contact (within one metre) with the infected patient.
- When working in a cohort bay it is acceptable to wear the same mask for the duration of the time spent in that bay, remembering that it must be changed if it becomes moist, damaged or contaminated.
- For all aerosol generating procedures (see Box 2) an FFP3 respirator mask, fluid-repellent gown, gloves and goggles or a full face visor should be worn by those performing the procedure and all others in the room.

Box 2   Aerosol-generating procedures

The procedures listed here are likely to generate an aerosol of the patient's secretions and can lead to transmission of infection where the patient undergoing the procedure has a respiratory tract infection.

- Intubation.
- Extubation.
- Manual ventilation.
- Open suctioning (oro/nasopharyngeal).
- Cardiopulmonary resuscitation.
- Bronchoscopy.
- Surgery and post mortem procedures in which high-speed devices are used.
- Non-invasive ventilation: bilevel positive airway pressure ventilation; continuous positive airway pressure ventilation; high-frequency oscillatory ventilation.
- Induction of sputum.

These procedures should only be performed when essential, should be carried out in a well-ventilated single room (preferably a negative pressure room) with the door closed and only those who are needed to undertake the procedure should be present.

Performing aerosol generating procedures in an open or communal patient area carries a high risk of transmission of infection for all those in the area for the duration of the procedure and for at least two hours afterwards.

- Staff required to wear an FFP3 respirator mask should be fit tested beforehand.
- Staff concerned about their exposure to the risk of infection via an incorrectly worn FFP3 should contact the local Occupational Health and Wellbeing Team for a review.
- Gloves and aprons are single-use items and must be changed between patients.
- Gloves, aprons, visors and masks worn in isolation rooms/cohort bays should be applied in the following order before entering the area:
  1. Apron/gown
  2. Mask
  3. Goggles
  4. Gloves
- Gloves, aprons, visors and masks worn in isolation rooms/cohort bays should be removed in the following order before leaving the area:

1. Gloves
2. Apron/ gown
3. Goggles
4. Mask

HAND HYGIENE   Hands must be washed immediately after removal of gloves, aprons, visors and masks. If hands are visibly clean, alcohol handrub can be used. If hands are soiled or contaminated, they must be washed with soap and water.

EQUIPMENT

• Equipment should be allocated to the individual patient or to a cohort of patients.
• Reusable equipment must be cleaned after each use.
• Fans should not be used as they disperse microorganisms throughout the environment.

THE ENVIRONMENT

• Isolation rooms/cohort bays should be cleaned at least once per day.
• Surfaces that are touched frequently, such as lockers, bed tables, toilets, toilet flush handles, taps, wash hand basins, door knobs and the area surrounding the patient, should be cleaned more frequently than once per day.
• Frequently touched surfaces should be cleaned immediately upon completion of an aerosol-generating procedure, as they will have become contaminated during the procedure. It will be necessary for nursing staff to do this whilst wearing the FFP3 mask, as domestic staff are not fit tested for FFP3 masks and their entry to this environment at this time would expose them to the risk of infection.
• Following an aerosol-generating procedure a minimum period of two hours should be allowed to elapse before domestic staff enter to undertake general environmental cleaning. This is required to allow the concentration of infectious particles in the air to reduce to a minimum in order to avoid exposing domestic staff to the risk of infection.
• The environment should be kept clean and free from clutter in order to make cleaning easier and to reduce the number of items that could become contaminated.
• Disposable cloths and detergent should be used for cleaning – disinfection is not required.
• Upon discharge/transfer of the patient, the room should be terminally cleaned in accordance with local policy. Cleaning is sufficient – disinfection is not required.

LINEN AND LAUNDRY

• Treat all used linen as 'infectious' and place in a red bag.

VISITORS

• The number of visitors should be kept to a minimum and visitors should adopt the same precautions as staff in terms of wearing gloves, aprons and masks and washing hands.
• Visitors to patients ventilated with non-invasive ventilation or high-frequency oscillatory ventilation may be exposed to the risk of infection during visiting and should be made aware of this.

Respiratory hygiene/cough etiquette (Catch it, Bin it, Kill it)

A disposable, single-use tissue should be used to cover the mouth and nose during coughing, sneezing, wiping or blowing noses. This should be discarded into a clinical waste bag and the hands should then be washed. Hands should always be washed after coughing, sneezing and using tissues. It may be necessary to help older people and children with respiratory hygiene.

Enteric precautions

Enteric precautions are required to minimise the risk of transmission of infection of diarrhoea and vomiting illnesses. Enteric precautions are as follows:

Hand washing

When patients have diarrhoea and vomiting, soap and water should be used to wash the hands. Alcohol handrubs are not reliable against all causes of diarrhoea and vomiting and should therefore not be used at these times.

Disposal of items contaminated with vomit and faeces

Ideally the patient should have their own designated flushable toilet, such as an en suite toilet in an isolation room. Where this is not possible the patient should be provided with a commode that is dedicated for their use only. After each use the commode should be cleaned with detergent and water then disinfected with a hypochlorite solution at 1000 parts per million available chlorine or cleaned and disinfected in one with a chlorine-based detergent at 1000 parts per million available chlorine. Those caring for the patient must use disposable gloves and aprons and wash their hands thoroughly after removal using soap and water.

Soiled/contaminated clothing and bed linen

Faeces should be removed from clothing and bedding and either flushed down the sluice hopper or discarded via a macerator or clinical waste bag. Disposal into a toilet can be used as a last resort but is best avoided due to the risk of splashing.

If visitors or relatives are taking soiled items home for laundering they should be advised to wash them at 60 °C or the hottest temperature that the fabric can tolerate. There is no need to use disinfectants or to soak items – washing in detergent is sufficient providing the washing machine is not overloaded in order to allow adequate dilution of microorganisms in the detergent and water.

Disinfection

Areas frequently touched after using the toilet such as the toilet itself, the toilet seat, the flush handle, the wash hand basin, taps, the door handle and the light switch should be disinfected daily and after each use using hypochlorite solution at 1000 parts per million available chlorine (see the subsection on management of blood and body fluids spillages and splashes).

Disposable bedpans and urinals should be discarded via a macerator. If disposable products are not available, the bedpan or urinal should be emptied into a sluice hopper and then cleaned and disinfected by one of the following methods:

- Wash with detergent and water and then disinfect with a hypochlorite solution at 1000 parts per million available chlorine.
- Use a chlorine-based detergent at 1000 parts per million available chlorine strength to clean and disinfect in one step.
- Place into a washer disinfector and allow a wash/disinfect cycle to complete.

Reusable bedpans and urinals can be emptied into the toilet but this is best avoided due to the risk of splashing.

Other considerations

- Hospital staff who have diarrhoea and vomiting illness should not be at work and should stay off until 48 hours after their last episode of diarrhoea and/or vomiting because they can still pass on the infection until this time.
- Hospital staff who prepare or serve food should not do so when they have diarrhoea and vomiting illness, as this can lead to transmission of infection.
- Visitors should be advised not to come to the hospital to visit when they have diarrhoea and vomiting, as they could easily pass it on.

Safe sharps practice, including sharps and splash injury management

Sharps are items (or parts of items) that could cause a laceration or a puncture wound. Table 5 sets out what is sharps waste and what is not.

Table 5 What is and what is not sharps waste

Sharps waste	Not sharps waste
• Needles	• Syringe bodies, other than the needle
• The needle part of a syringe	• Opened ampoules
• Scalpels, knives and other blades	• Tubes or tablets
• The patient end of an infusion set	• Swabs and dressings
• Nails	• Broken crockery and glass from non-healthcare items,
• Broken glass ampoules	e.g. coffee jar
	• Medicinal waste in the form of bottles, vials, ampoules, opened ampoules

Safe sharps practice
SHARPS CONTAINERS

• Ensure the sharps containers used in your clinical area are of a suitable size for the needs of the department, e.g. small portable containers in ward areas, limb bins in theatres and so on.
• Ensure that sharps containers are the correct colour for the type of sharps they are to be used for:
  ○ Yellow body and yellow lid for sharps containing any residue of medicinal products, but NOT cytotoxics/cytostatics.
  ○ Yellow body and purple lid for sharps containing cytotoxics/cytostatics.
  ○ Yellow body and orange lid for fully discharged sharps not containing any medicinal products.
• Ensure sharps containers are properly assembled with the lid securely attached all the way around. To do this properly it might be necessary to put the container on the floor and put your weight behind it.
• If a sharps container lid cannot be fitted properly (and sharp items have already been placed inside it) place the container inside a larger container and attach the lid.
• When assembling square sharps containers place the container on the floor and push down on diagonally opposite corners until an audible 'click' is heard.
• After assembling a sharps container, sign and date the label on the front and add the name of the hospital/ward in the relevant areas – this is a legal requirement. It denotes the date that the sharps container was first used (sharps containers should ideally be disposed of three months after first use) and gives an indication of the type of sharps waste contained therein.
• Store sharps containers at waist level or above to keep them out of the reach of children and to allow users to see how full they are, which will reduce the risk of sharps injuries associated with overfilled bins. Sharps containers should also be stored below shoulder height to avoid the risk of the container being pulled down from a height and spilling the contents over a person.
• Use the temporary closure mechanism on the sharps container to close the aperture when it is not in use.

- Do not overfill sharps containers – fill to the 'fill level' line only and then seal.
- Sign and date the label on the front of the container at the time that it is locked.
- Only discard sharps items into sharps containers; no domestic or clinical waste should be discarded in a sharps container.

SAFE HANDLING OF SHARPS

- Take all sharp items to the patient on a tray/trolley.
- Take a sharps container to the patient (to the point of care).
- Discard used sharps straight into a sharps container immediately after use.
- Do not separate needles from syringes – discard them as one unit.
- Do not resheathe needles – if this is essential use a resheathing device or place the cap on a flat surface and push the needle into it. Do not hold the needle in one hand and attempt to resheathe it with the other – this carries the risk of sharps injury.
- Do not carry sharps by hand or pass sharp items to another person.
- Do not remove scalpel blades by hand; use a blade-removing device or the notch on the sharps container (some sharps containers have notches on the lid – the smooth notch is for hands-free blade removal, while the stepped notch is for hands-free needle removal).

Sharps injury management

In the event of a sharps injury (needle pricks, cuts, scratches and bites) take the following steps:

1. Bleed it: encourage a few drops of blood to flow from the injured area by gently milking it – do not suck, scrub or squeeze it.
2. Wash it: wash the injured area thoroughly under running water with soap.
3. Cover it: apply a waterproof dressing to cover the puncture site.
4. Report it: immediately attend Occupational Health and Wellbeing if the injury is sustained during their opening hours; at other times attend the Emergency Department in case post-exposure prophylaxis is required.
5. Inform your line manager of your injury.
6. Complete an incident report form.

Note that post-exposure prophylaxis must be commenced within an hour of the injury for the best possible outcome to be achieved.

The following steps should also be taken:

- Try to obtain the following details of the patient the needle/ blade was used on before sustaining the injury (name, date of birth, phone number, doctor).
- If possible, inform the patient that they may be contacted after you have been risk assessed. It may be necessary for the patient to have a blood sample taken, for which their consent is required. Occupational Health should organise this with the patient's doctor, follow up the result and coordinate any further action that is required.

Splash injury management

In the event of a blood/body fluid splash to the eyes/mouth or on to broken skin:

1. Rinse the affected area with plenty of running water – do not swallow.
2. Immediately attend Occupational Health and Wellbeing if the injury is sustained during their opening hours; at other times attend the Emergency Department in case post-exposure prophylaxis is required.
3. Inform your line manager of your injury.
4. Complete an incident report form.

Safe disposal of clinical waste

This section discusses waste segregation and disposal and includes sections on Category A pathogens and cytostatic and cytotoxic drugs.

Careful waste disposal and appropriate segregation are important for infection control and the environment. Disposal of clinical waste is more expensive than domestic waste disposal and therefore careful waste segregation can save money.

Segregation of waste is required by law; failure to adhere to waste management legislation can have repercussions for the organisation in terms of financial penalty or loss of reputation. Everyone has a responsibility to segregate waste properly at the point of disposal. Clinical, domestic and sharps waste must be segregated wherever they are stored prior to final disposal.

Waste segregation and disposal

WASTE SACK HOLDERS Waste sack holders should be placed as close as possible to where the waste is generated to allow prompt disposal. In clinical areas waste sack holders should fully encase the waste sack and be fire-retardant, with a foot-operable lid to allow hands-free opening and closure. Domestic waste bins should be placed next to hand wash-basins in order that paper towels are disposed of correctly and clinical waste bins should ideally be placed in areas not accessed by visitors.

WASTE CATEGORIES AND COLOUR CODING Table 6 discusses waste types and the colour of waste sack/sharps container they should be placed in.

Table 6 Waste categories and colour coding of waste sacks

Colour	Description and contents
Yellow	Highly infectious clinical waste:
	• anatomical waste (see red containers below)
	• chemically contaminated samples and diagnostic kits
	• medicinally contaminated infectious waste
	• contaminated with Category A pathogens (see below)
Orange	Infectious clinical waste such as dressings and items contaminated with blood and body fluids
Purple	Cytotoxic and cytostatic waste (see full list of medicines below)
Yellow and black	Offensive/hygiene waste such as catheter and stoma bags, sanitary towels and tampons, incontinence pads, babies nappies, uncontaminated (used) gloves and aprons
Red	Anatomical waste, including recognisable body parts and placentae
Black/clear	Domestic waste such as flowers, newspapers, wrappers, paper towels
Blue	Medicinal waste
White	Amalgam waste

ADDITIONAL CONSIDERATIONS

• Liquid waste, such as blood, should have a gelling agent added to it before it is placed into a clinical waste sack to avoid the risk of spillage.
• Waste sacks must be no more than three-quarters full when sealed.
• Waste sacks should be sealed using a ratchet tag and the swan-neck method (see Figure 3).

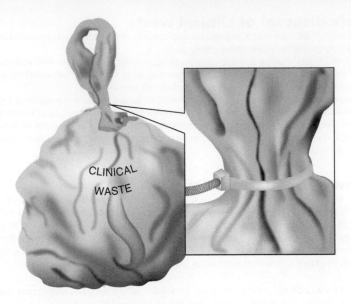

Figure 3   The swan-neck method

Method:

1. Remove the waste sack from the sack holder when no more than three-quarters full.
2. Twist the neck of the sack.
3. Fold the twisted neck of the sack over on itself to form a loop.
4. Secure the loop close to the base of the twist using a ratchet tie.
5. Place the secured waste sack into a rigid clinical waste container.

Category A pathogens

Bacillus anthracis (cultures only)
Brucella abortus (cultures only)
Brucella melitensis (cultures only)
Brucella suis (cultures only)
Burkholderia mallei – *Pseudomonas mallei* – Glanders (cultures only)
Burkholderia pseudomallei – *Pseudomonas pseudomallei* (cultures only)
Chlamydia psittaci – avian strains (cultures only)
Clostridium botulinum (cultures only)
Coccidioides immitis (cultures only)
Coxiella burnetii (cultures only)
Crimean–Congo haemorrhagic fever virus
Dengue virus (cultures only)
Eastern equine encephalitis virus (cultures only)
Escherichia coli, verotoxigenic (cultures only)
Ebola virus
Flexal virus
Francisella tularensis (cultures only)

Guanarito virus
Hantaan virus
Hantavirus causing haemorrhagic fever with renal syndrome
Hendra virus
Hepatitis B virus (cultures only)
Herpes B virus (cultures only)
Human immunodeficiency virus (cultures only)
Highly pathogenic avian influenza virus (cultures only)
Japanese encephalitis virus (cultures only)
Junin virus
Kyasanur Forest disease virus
Lassa virus
Machupo virus
Marburg virus
Monkeypox virus
Mycobacterium tuberculosis (cultures only)
Nipah virus
Omsk haemorrhagic fever virus
Poliovirus (cultures only)
Rabies virus (cultures only)
Rickettsia prowazekii (cultures only)
Rickettsia rickettsii (cultures only)
Rift Valley fever virus (cultures only)
Russian spring–summer encephalitis virus (cultures only)
Sabia virus
Shigella dysenteriae type 1 (cultures only)
Tick-borne encephalitis virus (cultures only)
Variola virus
Venezuelan equine encephalitis virus (cultures only)
West Nile virus (cultures only)
Yellow fever virus (cultures only)
Yersinia pestis (cultures only)

Cytotoxic/cytostatic drugs
This list is not exhaustive and may not include all very new, unlicensed or trial medicines.

NEW LIST OF NON-CHEMOTHERAPY CYTOTOXIC/CYTOSTATIC DRUGS
Anastrozole
Azathioprine
Bicalutamide
Chloramphenicol – classified as a category 2A carcinogen and as such will include eyedrops with a concentration of 0.1% (the legal threshold in waste legislation)
Ciclosporin, Cidofovir, Coal tar containing products Colchicine
Danazol
Diethylstilbestrol
Dinoprostone
Dithranol containing products
Dutasteride
Estradiol
Exemestane
Finasteride

Flutamide
Ganciclovir
Gonadotrophin, chorionic
Goserelin
Interferon containing products (including peginterferon)
Leflunomide
Letrozole
Leuprorelin acetate
Medroxyprogesterone
Megestrol
Menotropins
Mifepristone
Mycophenolate mofetil
Nafarelin
Oestrogen containing products
Oxytocin (including syntocinon and syntometrine)
Podophyllyn
Progesterone containing products
Raloxifene
Ribavarin
Sirolimus
Streptozocin
Tacrolimus
Tamoxifen
Testosterone
Thalidomide
Toremifene
Trifluridine
Triptorelin
Valganciclovir
Zidovudine

Cancer chemotherapy drugs
Aldesleukin
Alemtuzumab
Amsacrine
Arsenic trioxide
Asparaginase
Bleomycin
Bortezomib
Busulphan
Capecitabine
Carboplatin
Carmustine
Cetuximab
Chlorambucil
Cisplatin
Cladribine
Cyclophosphamide
Cytarabine
Dacarbazine

Dactinomycin
Daunorubicin
Dasatinib
Docetaxel
Doxorubicin
Epirubicin
Estramustine
Etoposide
Fludarabine
Fluorouracil
Gemcitabine
Gemtuzumab
Hydroxycarbamide
Idarubicin
Ifosfamide
Imatinib mesylate
Irinotecan
Lomustine
Melphalan
Mercaptopurine
Methotrexate
Mitomycin
Mitotane
Mitoxantrone
Oxaliplatin
Paclitaxel
Pentamidine
Pentostatin
Procarbazine
Raltitrexed
Rituximab
Temozolomide
Thiotepa
Topotecan
Trastuzumab
Vidaradine
Vinblastine
Vincristine

Safe handling of linen and laundry

Linen must be handled and stored in such a way as to prevent clean linen from becoming contaminated and dirty linen from causing contamination of hands, surfaces and clean linen. Used linen must be laundered effectively to render it clean and free from blood and body fluids, stains and contamination.

Clean linen storage

Clean linen should be stored in a clean, designated area that is not used for anything else. Ideally this should be a closed cupboard, which should not be used to store other items in order to avoid linen becoming dirty or contaminated.

If no dedicated cupboards are available and linen is stored on a trolley or shelving in a corridor it should be covered to prevent contamination and accumulation of dust. The cover must be waterproof and able to withstand cleaning and disinfection.

Linen should be taken from the designated storage area as needed, extra items should not be stored in patient areas, as they may become contaminated and become a vehicle for transmission of infection. This is particularly important during outbreaks of infection; extra linen stored in cupboards and on trolleys in patient areas should be removed and sent for laundering.

Clean linen found to be stained or damaged should not be used but should also not be destroyed or sent for laundering. It should be returned in the reject bag to the laundry facility. Laundry facilities carry out repairs on damaged items that have small tears – it is important not to make tears of holes larger as this will render them unfit for repair, which may result in the hospital being charged for a replacement.

Used linen

Always take a linen buggy/skip to the bedside when changing beds in order that used and/or soiled linen can be placed directly into it. This reduces the possibility of contamination of surfaces from the used linen.

Used linen should never be placed on the floor or on locker tops, bed tables, radiators, window sills or any surface other than in the linen buggy/skip or on the integral bed shelf at the end of the bed.

Used linen should not be shaken once it has been taken off the bed, as this will disperse skin scales and debris into the air.

Once used linen has been bagged it should not be handled again by anyone (hospital laundry facilities have systems to avoid used linen from being handled manually).

Infectious linen

Linen used with a patient known or suspected to have an infection, or that has become contaminated with blood or other body fluids, should be placed directly into a colour-coded bag that identifies it as infected/soiled linen. Red bags are often used (sometimes water-soluble bags are used to avoid any handling at the laundry facility) – follow local policy for colour-coding guidance. This bag should then be sealed and placed into the linen cart.

Linen that is heavily soiled or stained and unlikely to be cleaned effectively should be disposed of as clinical waste.

Storage of used linen

Used linen should be removed from clinical areas regularly to avoid it accumulating in the dirty utility room. After removal from the clinical area it should be stored in a designated storage area, which is secure and inaccessible to the public.

Asepsis and aseptic non-touch technique

Asepsis is the freedom from contamination by pathogenic organisms. The aim of asepsis is to avoid introducing microorganisms to a susceptible site, such as a wound, or the insertion site of a medical device, such as an intravenous cannula.

Aseptic non-touch technique (ANTT)

The aseptic non-touch technique is a standardised approach that supports clinical staff to maintain asepsis in clinical practice by identifying 'key parts' and 'key sites' to protect them from contamination.

KEY PARTS   These are the vital parts of clinical equipment that come into direct or indirect contact with key sites and any active key parts connected to the patient and any liquid infusion. If these parts become contaminated they present a significant risk of infection.

KEY SITES   Key sites are open wounds and medical device access sites.

Standard and surgical ANTT

There are two approaches in ANTT – standard and surgical. The choice of approach is dependent on a risk assessment of the technical difficulty of the procedure.

STANDARD ANTT   Standard ANTT is suitable for technically simple procedures that are short in duration, have a small key site and few key parts. A main general aseptic field is maintained and a microaseptic field is used around the key site and key parts. Non-sterile gloves are worn. Standard ANTT can be used for intravenous cannulation, intravenous therapy, urinary catheterisation and simple wound dressings.

SURGICAL ANTT   Surgical ANTT is used for complicated procedures that take an extended period of time, have large open key sites and numerous key parts. A main aseptic field is used with critical microaseptic fields. Sterile gloves are worn and a non-touch technique is used where practical. Surgical ANTT is used for surgery, insertion of central lines (peripheral and central) and large or complex wound dressings.

OTHER THINGS TO CONSIDER   Ward cleaning should have ceased before embarking upon an ANTT and the privacy curtains should be drawn in advance in order to allow dust to settle before exposing the key site.

Clean wounds should be dressed before dirty wounds, wounds should be exposed for as short a time as possible and skin should be clean before an ANTT is started.

FOOTNOTE   At the time of writing this book new guidance and materials on 'The ANTT-Approach' were anticipated from www.ANTT.org.uk.

3 Wider Aspects

Managing an outbreak of infection

This section is broken down into the following subsections: definitions, patient management, communication, and staff, visitors and others.

Definitions

An *outbreak of infection* is two or more people infected with the same organism that have something else in common, such as their location or the timing of their symptoms. The term 'outbreak' is also used when the observed number of people infected with a particular organism in a particular location is greater than the number expected.

A *suspected outbreak of infection* is two or more people having similar symptoms in the same clinical area but where the cause is not yet established, e.g. two patients in the same bay with diarrhoea and vomiting.

An outbreak of infection is considered a *major outbreak* when there are a large number of people infected or the infection is caused by a notifiable disease or the infection is a health hazard to the local population. The infection control doctor will decide if an outbreak is a major outbreak.

Patient management

ISOLATION OF SYMPTOMATIC PATIENTS Symptomatic patients should be isolated with isolation precautions implemented. If isolation facilities are not available, the area(s) where the patients are being cared for should be closed to admissions, transfers and discharges, with isolation precautions implemented. Movement of patients at this stage is not advisable and may expose more patients (and staff) to the risk of infection. Contact the infection control team and bed manager for advice.

IDENTIFYING THE CAUSE Take the relevant samples or swabs from the patient for microbiological testing to determine the cause of the suspected outbreak. If you are unclear about the samples that are required contact the microbiology laboratory for advice. Timing of samples is important; the sooner a sample is taken, the earlier the cause of the infection is known, which makes managing the risks of transmission simpler.

SCREENING It may be necessary to screen other patients in the same ward/clinical area to ascertain if they have been infected with the causative organism. The infection control doctor will advise on this.

IDENTIFYING THE SOURCE It may be necessary to examine clinical practice – the cleaning and disinfection techniques used for instruments, equipment and the environment; theatre discipline and kitchen hygiene, etc. – to determine the source of the

Rapid Infection Control Nursing, First Edition. Shona Ross and Sarah Furrows.
© 2014 John Wiley & Sons, Ltd. Published 2014 by John Wiley & Sons, Ltd.

infection. The infection control team will lead on this and liaise with contractors and external agencies as required.

CLOSED BAYS AND WARDS   The infection control team and bed managers will manage beds, movement of patients, transfers and discharges throughout the outbreak.

ADMISSIONS, TRANSFERS AND DISCHARGES   Admissions to the ward and transfers and discharges to other wards, care homes and hospitals will be restricted during an outbreak, if not stopped altogether. This will depend on the cause of the outbreak and the infection control team will advise on this.

PATIENT TRANSFER   Transferring a patient from a ward closed due to an outbreak of infection can lead to a further outbreak in the receiving area, even if the patient is asymptomatic, as they could be incubating the infection.

If it is necessary to transfer an infected patient (or a patient without symptoms from an area affected by an outbreak of infection) to another ward/hospital/department, it is essential to inform staff at the receiving area of the outbreak situation in your ward before the transfer takes place in order that they can take the necessary isolation precautions when the patient arrives. This can be done by phone prior to the transfer. Details of the patient's infectious status should be documented in their notes and discussed at handover. No infected/infectious patient should ever be transferred without prior notice to the receiving area. Patients with diarrhoea should not be transferred unless it is an emergency situation.

If the transfer will involve patient transfer or ambulance staff they too should be informed prior to the transfer. Ideally, this patient should go last on their list, providing it is medically safe for the patient to wait until then. The ambulance/patient transport vehicle should be cleaned and disinfected once the transfer is complete.

Gloves and an apron should be worn by staff involved in assisting the patient out of bed on to a trolley or into a chair and should then be removed and the hands washed. Gloves and aprons should not be worn when moving a patient between wards/departments.

DOCUMENTATION   It is essential that the following information is recorded for each patient with symptoms:

1. Name.
2. Date of birth.
3. Date and time of onset of symptoms.
4. Date and time symptoms resolved.
5. Dates and times of samples sent for testing.
6. Results of microbiology tests.
7. Date of admission.
8. Where they were admitted from, e.g. home, a care home, another hospital.
9. Have they been in contact with anyone else with similar symptoms?
10. Stool charts should be maintained when patients have diarrhoea. It is important to record the time, nature and frequency of bowel movements, using the same terminology. The Bristol stool form scale is useful for this.

IDENTIFYING CONTACTS   It may be necessary to identify individuals who have been in contact with those who are infected. The infection control team will manage this.

DISCHARGE HOME   For some conditions it is acceptable for patients to be discharged to their own home. This should be discussed with the infection control team before making any arrangements to move the patient.

POST-OUTBREAK CLEANING AND DISINFECTION   At the end of the outbreak, before any new patients are admitted, the clinical area must be cleaned and disinfected with detergent followed by a chlorine-releasing agent at 1000 parts per million available chlorine strength, or cleaned and disinfected in one step using a chlorine-based detergent at 1000 parts per million available chlorine strength. Curtains must also be changed.

Communication

Rapid detection of an outbreak is crucial in controlling the numbers of those who are exposed and become infected. If you suspect an outbreak in your place of work you should report it immediately in order that you receive the support you need to manage it and minimise the risk of further spread.

The following list of people is whom you should contact – if you cannot get the first person you call, try the next one on the list. You do not need to contact each person listed; you just need to inform one of them in order that they can get involved with managing the situation and notify senior managers and directors if the operation of the hospital or provision of services is likely to be affected.

1. Ward manager (if that is not you)
2. The infection control team (outside office hours, contact the on-call microbiologist)
3. On-call manager (if the outbreak occurs at a weekend Matrons and Head of Nursing will not be available)
4. Matron
5. Bed manager
6. Head of Nursing
7. Divisional Manager
8. Divisional Director
9. Director of Nursing
10. Chief Operating Officer
11. Chief Executive Officer

The hospital cleaning manager must also be informed of the outbreak to allow preparation to be made for increased cleaning throughout the outbreak.

After initial escalation and reporting it is important to ensure that all staff are aware of the outbreak and of the isolation precautions to take. The infection control team will inform external agencies such as the local Health Protection Unit and the Consultant in Communicable Disease Control (CCDC) and convene outbreak meetings as required.

NOTIFIABLE DISEASES   If the cause of the outbreak is a notifiable disease the medical staff responsible for the patient must complete the 'notification of infection diseases' documentation and submit it to the local health protection unit.

DECLARING THE OUTBREAK OVER   The infection control team will declare the outbreak over when there are no new cases and the incubation period for new cases of the causative organism has elapsed.

MEDIA ENQUIRIES   There may be enquiries from the media about the outbreak, particularly if a large number of people are affected, if it is caused by something of a sensitive nature (such as scabies) or an unusual organism, or if a concerned patient, relative or visitor contacts a journalist. You should not discuss the outbreak with the media; you should advise them to contact the communication team in accordance with local policy.

POST-OUTBREAK LEARNING   Any lessons learned during and from the outbreak should be discussed with the whole team involved. The infection control team will lead on this with support from the local Health Protection Unit.

Staff, visitors and others

RESTRICTING STAFF MOVEMENT   Ideally, the staff working in a closed ward/bay should remain in that area and not work elsewhere in order to minimise the risk of transmitting the infection to others.

STAFF WHO BECOME INFECTED   It is important to record the following details for members of staff who become infected:

1. Name.
2. Date of birth.
3. Date and time of onset of symptoms.
4. Date and time symptoms resolved.
5. Dates and times of samples sent for testing.
6. Results of microbiology tests.
7. Clinical areas where they worked prior to the onset of symptoms.
8. Were they in contact with anyone else with similar symptoms, or any patients identified as part of an outbreak?

The Occupational Health team will collect this information.

MINIMISING THE RISK TO OTHERS   During an outbreak of infection it is important to expose as few people as possible to the risk of infection. For that reason, the following precautions apply:

- There should be no maintenance work, repairs or renovations in the affected area until the outbreak is over, unless urgent or essential.
- The affected area should not be used as a thoroughfare to access other wards or departments.
- Visitors should be restricted and children should be excluded from visiting until the outbreak is over.
- Adults and children should not visit the hospital when they have diarrhoea and/or vomiting.
- Children should not visit the hospital during outbreaks of diarrhoea and vomiting.

Isolation and screening of contacts

In the event that a patient in close proximity to other patients, i.e. in the same bay, is diagnosed as being colonised or infected with a resistant organism, it may be necessary to implement isolation precautions and screen the other patients for the presence of the organism.

The rationale for this is that the patients in the bay have been exposed to the risk of becoming infected with the organism. Implementation of isolation precautions and screening of the exposed patients for the organism allows a degree of control over the potential spread of the organism in addition to treatment of those who test positive.

A good example to use here is methicillin-resistant *Staphylococcus aureus* (MRSA). If a patient in a six-bedded bay in a surgical ward tested positive for MRSA, the other patients in the bay would be screened for MRSA and isolation precautions would be implemented. Isolation precautions would remain in place until all results were known. Other patients found to be MRSA positive would be isolated and treated and those who were negative would no longer require isolation precautions.

Local practice on the isolation of contacts will vary from place to place. This practice is common for alert organisms, which includes the following:

- Multiresistant *Acinetobacter baumanii* (MRAB)
- Extended spectrum beta lactamase (ESBLs) and other antibiotic-resistant bacteria
- *Clostridium difficile*
- Diarrhoeal infections
- Glycopeptide (Vancomycin)-resistant *Enterococci*
- MRSA
- Panton–Valentine leukocidin (PVL) associated *Staphylococcus aureus*
- Respiratory viruses
- Tuberculosis
- Viral haemorrhagic fevers

Please check with your local infection control team for the organisms that require isolation and screening of contacts in your organisation.

Your health and wellbeing

As a healthcare worker there are a number of things you can do to protect yourself from the risk of harm and infection and to present yourself professionally at work. Please note that MRSA screening for staff is not currently recommended by the Department of Health.

You must not come to work if you have an unexplained rash or diarrhoea and should contact the local occupational health and/or infection control teams for further advice. In diarrhoeal illness you should not return to work until you have been free from diarrhoea for 48 hours.

Maternity workers should not work clinically whilst they have a cold sore and should explore the possibility of temporary redeployment as an interim measure.

Personal hygiene
- It is regarded as good practice to wear a clean uniform every day.
- Nails should be short, clean and free from nail varnish, false nails and nail attachments.
- No hand or wrist jewellery other than a plain metal band should be worn whilst caring for patients.

Laundering uniforms
Uniforms should be laundered at 60 °C. It is important not to overfill the washing machine, as dilution of microorganisms with water and detergent is required for cleansing and disinfection to occur. The type of detergent used is not important.

The Occupational Health and Wellbeing department

The Occupational Health team are there to promote and maintain your mental and physical wellbeing, which involves pre-placement screening of all new employees for infectious diseases such as tuberculosis.

EXPOSURE-PRONE PROCEDURES   Healthcare workers who perform exposure-prone procedures are required to provide current UK validated evidence that they have tested negative for hepatitis B surface antigen, hepatitis C antibody and HIV antibody. Those returning to the NHS following a sabbatical or time spent abroad must attend the local occupational health department for assessment of the risk of BBV infection having been acquired. To decline these tests would preclude a healthcare worker from performing exposure-prone procedures, as would a positive HIV test. A positive test for hepatitis B surface antigen (HBsAg) or hepatitis C antibody (HCAb) would necessitate further testing.

COMMUNICABLE DISEASES   Healthcare workers exposed to a serious communicable disease are obliged to seek professional advice about the need to be tested.

IMMUNITY ASSESSMENT   Upon commencement of a healthcare worker role in the NHS you will be assessed for immunity to the following:

- Hepatitis B
- Chicken pox (Varicella zoster)
- Measles
- Mumps
- Rubella

A healthcare worker who has no evidence of prior immunity and refuses to be vaccinated against measles, mumps, rubella and varicella is at risk of infection and subsequently provides an infection risk to patients, other staff and close contacts, which may have an impact upon their ability to function in their chosen role.

The deceased

Safe handling and disposal of the body after death is important when the deceased was known or suspected to have an infection. It is also important to bear in mind the risk of undiagnosed infection. A person who was considered infectious in life may remain infectious after death. The following infections and pathogens are a particular risk to those handling the recently deceased:

- Tuberculosis
- Hepatitis B
- Hepatitis C
- HIV
- Gastrointestinal organisms
- Group A streptococcal infection
- Transmissible spongiform encephalopathies agents such as Creutzfeldt–Jakob disease
- Meningitis
- Septicaemia (particularly meningococcal)

The risk of transmission of infection can be avoided by applying the standard principles of infection prevention and control at all times, regardless of any known or perceived risk. Table 7 contains guidance for handling cadavers with infections.

Body bags

In addition to the guidance given in Table 7, body bags should be used if there is any risk of leakage of blood or body fluids, for badly damaged bodies and for those with a high risk of being infectious, e.g. intravenous drug users.

Handling high-risk bodies on the ward

- Minimal handling of the deceased is advisable.
- Cover any cuts or grazes you have on your hands or arms with a waterproof dressing.
- Any injury sustained by you during last offices should be managed as for sharps/splash injuries and reported as a clinical incident.
- If a family member or attendant is involved in preparing the body (as part of their culture) they must be informed of the infection risks and protection measures required before touching the body and must adopt the same protective measures as staff.
- Those who handle the deceased, including family members and porters, should wear gloves and an apron.
- If there is any risk of splashing to the face during last offices, a surgical mask and eye protection should also be worn.
- Cover all wounds and breaks in the skin of the deceased (including insertion sites of indwelling devices such as intravenous cannulae that are removed during last offices) with a waterproof dressing.
- Take a sharps container to the bedside to allow disposal of sharps straight into the sharps container.
- Gloves and aprons must be discarded as clinical waste immediately after removal. Portering staff should follow the guidance in Box 3.
- Hands must be washed after removing gloves and aprons.
- Mortuary staff must be informed of the infection status of the deceased before transfer from ward to mortuary takes place.
- Follow local policy on labelling of the body prior to transfer to the mortuary.

Table 7   Guidance for handling cadavers with infections

Degree of risk	Infection	Body bag required	Visiting, viewing, touching allowed
Low (notifiable)	Acute encephalitis	No	Yes
	Leprosy	No	Yes
	Measles	No	Yes
	Meningitis (except meningococcal)	No	Yes
	Mumps	No	Yes
	Rubella	No	Yes
	Tetanus	No	Yes
	Whooping cough	No	Yes
Low (not notifiable)	Chickenpox/shingles	No	Yes
	Cryptosporidiosis	No	Yes
	Dermatophytosis	No	Yes
	Legionellosis	No	Yes
	Lyme disease	No	Yes
	Psittacosis	No	Yes
	Methicillin-resistant *Staphylococcus aureus*	No	Yes
	Tetanus	No	Yes
Medium (notifiable)	Food poisoning	No/Adv	Yes
	Hepatitis A	No	Yes
	Acute poliomyelitis	No	Yes
	Diphtheria	Adv	Yes
	Dysentery	Adv	Yes
	Leptospirosis (Weil's disease)	No	Yes
	Malaria	No	Yes
	Meningococcal septicaemia (+/– meningitis)	Adv	Yes
	Paratyphoid fever	Adv	Yes
	Cholera	No	Yes
	Scarlet fever	Adv	Yes
	Tuberculosis	Adv	Yes
	Typhoid fever	Adv	Yes
	Typhus	Adv	No
Medium (not notifiable)	HIV/AIDS	Adv	Yes
	Q fever	No	Yes
High (notifiable)	Hepatitis B, C	Yes	Yes
High (not notifiable)	Transmissible spongiform encephalopathies agents such as Creutzfeldt–Jakob disease	Yes	No*
	Invasive group A streptococcal infection	Yes	No
High (rare) (notifiable)	Anthrax	Adv	No
	Plague	Yes	No
	Rabies	Yes	No
	Smallpox	Yes	No
	Viral haemorrhagic fever	Yes	No
	Yellow Fever	Yes	No

Adv = advisable and may be required by local health regulations.
*Viewing is not permitted if a post mortem examination has taken place.

Box 3   Guidance for porters

- Gloves and an apron should be worn when moving the deceased from the bed to the mortuary trolley, then removed and hands washed.
- Gloves and an apron do not need to be worn when pushing the mortuary trolley.
- Gloves and an apron should be worn when moving the deceased from the mortuary trolley to the body store, then removed and hands washed.

Specimen collection and storage

For accurate results to be obtained, specimens should be received by the laboratory as soon as possible and preferably within 24 hours. After this time the dominant or more virulent organisms (such as staphylococci) will flourish and the weaker organisms, e.g. anaerobes, will die off and a false result may be obtained.

Note that gonococci are not expected to survive in swabs for more than 18–24 hours.

Specimens should be refrigerated as shown in Table 8. In the absence of a specimen fridge, storage at room temperature is acceptable overnight *only where stated.* **All swabs not sent to the lab the same day should be refrigerated overnight. The laboratory will generally discard specimens over 48 hours old.**

Table 8 Specimen collection and storage

Specimen	Storage	Container	To lab
Wound swab	Refrigerate overnight if not reaching lab same day	Bacterial swab containing transport medium (usually black or blue top)	ASAP/within 24 hours
Viral swab	Refrigerate overnight if not reaching lab same day	Viral swab or viral transport medium	ASAP/within 24 hours
Chlamydia (1) First catch urine	Refrigerate overnight if not reaching lab same day.	Plain universal container or Chlamydia transport tube	ASAP/within 24 hours
Chlamydia (2) Female endocervical swab/ female self-taken low vaginal swab	Refrigerate overnight if not reaching lab same day	Chlamydia swab or Chlamydia transport tube	ASAP/within 24 hours
Tissue/pus	Refrigerate if not possible to send directly to lab	Plain universal container	Immediately
Urine	Refrigerate overnight only *If antibiotics are to be commenced immediately, obtain a specimen now and refrigerate until collection, even if at a weekend/public holiday*	Plain universal container	ASAP/within 24 hours
Sputum	Refrigerate overnight if not reaching lab same day	Plain universal container	ASAP/within 24 hours
Faeces	Refrigerate overnight if not reaching lab same day	Stool specimen container	ASAP/ within 24 hours
Blood cultures	**Send directly to lab for incubation**	Blood culture bottles	Immediately
Serology/Virology blood tests	Refrigerate overnight if not reaching lab same day	Serum or EDTA blood tube (check with laboratory, depends on the test required)	ASAP/within 24 hours
CSF	**Send directly to lab**	Plain universal container	Immediately

Audit

In infection control, audit is used to measure, monitor and report on standards of clinical practice and hygiene and environmental factors.

The audit cycle

The audit cycle has four stages (Figure 4), similar to the nursing process (assess, plan, implement, evaluate).

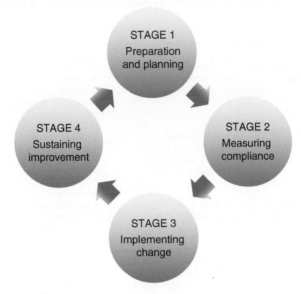

Figure 4   The audit cycle

It is important that the audit cycle is implemented and completed properly and not viewed merely as a 'ticking the box' exercise. It needs to be owned by those who deliver the care or provide the service that is being audited. Self-audit and peer audit are useful ways to measure your own practice standards.

Audit resources

In addition to existing tools available to you from the local infection control team, there are a number of resources available from the Department of Health and the Infection Prevention Society.

Department of Health

Best practice guidance, audit tools and resources on the following topics are available from The National Archives website (http://webarchive.nationalarchives.gov.uk/20120118164404/; http://hcai.dh.gov.uk/whatdoido/high-impact-interventions/):

- Creating a high-impact intervention
- Central venous catheters
- Peripheral intravenous cannula
- Renal haemodialysis care
- Prevention of surgical site infection
- Ventilator associated pneumonia
- Urinary catheter care
- *Clostridium difficile* infection
- Cleaning and decontamination
- Chronic wounds
- Enteral feeding
- Blood cultures

The Infection Prevention Society (IPS)

In addition to a dental audit tool, the IPS has developed a series of quality improvement tools (QIT) and rapid improvement tools (RIT), which are available to IPS members on the IPS website.

QIT should be used to measure compliance with practice and environmental standards to gather baseline information and highlight areas for improvement.

RIT should be used to highlight areas for improvement and assess whether planned changes were implemented.

QUALITY IMPROVEMENT TOOLS (QIT)

- Care setting tools:
  - Care homes
  - Endoscopy – decontamination
  - Endoscopy – environment
  - ECT treatment suite mental health
  - GP surgery/health centre
  - Hydrotherapy/swimming pool
  - In- and outpatient area departments
  - Inpatient/care home mental health/ learning sisabilities
  - Day/resource centre mental health/ learning disabilities
  - Operating theatres
  - Outpatients mental health/ learning disabilities
  - Transportation of specimens
  - Vaccine storage and transportation
  - Vehicles

- Clinical practice tools:
  - Asepsis
  - Central venous catheter (CVC) continuing care
  - Central venous catheter (CVC) insertion
  - Isolation precautions
  - Enteral feeding
  - Hand hygiene environment
  - Hand hygiene observation tool (5 moments) (use RIT)
  - Hand hygiene technique
  - Peripheral vascular device (PVD) continuing care
  - Peripheral vascular device (PVD) insertion
  - Scrub procedures
  - Standard precautions
  - Theatre asepsis
  - Urinary catheter insertion
  - Urinary catheter daily care

RAPID IMPROVEMENT TOOLS (RIT)

- Care setting tools:
  - Care homes
  - Endoscopy – decontamination
  - Endoscopy – environment
  - ECT treatment suite mental health
  - GP surgery/health centre
  - Hydrotherapy/swimming pool
  - In- and outpatient area departments
  - Inpatient/care home mental health/ learning disabilities
  - Day/resource centre
  - Operating theatres
  - Outpatients mental health/learning disabilities
  - Transportation of specimens
  - Vaccine storage and transportation
  - Vehicles

- Clinical practice tools:
  - Asepsis
  - Central venous catheter (CVC) continuing care
  - Central venous catheter (CVC) insertion
  - Isolation precautions
  - Enteral feeding
  - Hand hygiene environment
  - Hand hygiene observation tool (5 moments)
  - Hand hygiene technique
  - Peripheral vascular device (PVD) continuing care
  - Peripheral vascular device (PVD) insertion
  - Scrub procedures
  - Standard precautions
  - Theatre asepsis
  - Urinary catheter insertion
  - Urinary catheter daily care

Assistance dogs, ward pets and visiting animals

Some patients benefit greatly from being visited by an animal whilst in hospital and others rely on an assistance dog to attend for treatment. Animals can come into hospital premises providing the following guidance is adhered to.

Guide dogs, hearing dogs and assistance dogs

A person reliant on an assistance dog can bring the dog with them whenever they attend an outpatient appointment, but the dog cannot accompany the patient if they are admitted to the hospital as an inpatient. As such the patient may require an alternative means of support, which must be arranged before they are admitted. At the time of discharge it will be necessary to arrange for the assistance dog to be available at the time that the patient arrives home.

In very exceptional circumstances an assistance dog may be allowed to accompany the patient into hospital, but this must be discussed with the local infection control team before it is arranged.

Ward pets

Caged birds and rodents are not suitable as ward pets in the hospital setting due to the opportunity for contamination to occur via their bedding, fur and feathers.

Fish tanks in clinical areas must be maintained and cleaned as directed by an aquatics expert to minimise the risk of infection via contaminated water and to avoid harming the fish.

Visiting animals

Organised visits from agencies such as 'Pets as therapy dogs' (PAT dogs) should be discussed in advance with infection control before they are agreed to.

Visiting animals must be fully immunised and healthy on the day of the visit and restricted to non-clinical areas, e.g. the ward foyer or day room.

Special considerations for long-term or terminally ill patients should be discussed with infection control before a visit is arranged.

Visits to restricted areas should only take place in agreement with senior nursing staff for that area and the local infection control team. The following are restricted areas:

- ITU/ HDU/ CCU
- NNU
- Food preparation areas
- Patients in isolation
- Patients who are neutropenic or immunosuppressed

After contact with a visiting animal patients and staff must wash their hands.

If the animal passes urine or faeces during the visit this should be cleaned up using paper towels and detergent wipes, with gloves and an apron worn and hands washed immediately afterwards.

Notifiable diseases

In England and Wales, doctors have a statutory responsibility to notify the Consultant in Communicable Disease Control (CCDC) at the local Health Protection Unit or the 'Proper Officer' of the Local Authority of all suspected cases of the following infectious diseases:

- Acute encephalitis
- Acute infectious hepatitis
- Acute meningitis
- Acute poliomyelitis
- Anthrax
- Botulism
- Brucellosis
- Cholera
- Diphtheria
- Enteric fever (typhoid or paratyphoid fever)
- Food poisoning
- Haemolytic uraemic syndrome (HUS)
- Infectious bloody diarrhoea
- Invasive group A streptococcal disease
- Legionnaires' disease
- Leprosy
- Malaria
- Measles
- Meningococcal septicaemia
- Mumps
- Plague
- Rabies
- Rubella
- SARS
- Scarlet fever
- Smallpox
- Tetanus
- Tuberculosis
- Typhus
- Viral haemorrhagic fever (VHF)
- Whooping cough
- Yellow fever

Upon diagnosis of a suspected notifiable disease, the doctor attending the patient should complete a notification certificate. It is important not to wait for laboratory confirmation of the infection before notification. The certificate should be sent to the CCDC or the Proper Officer within three days. If the case is considered urgent the CCDC/ Proper Officer should be informed verbally within 24 hours. (Proper Officers are required to pass on the entire notification to the PHE within three days of a case being notified, or within 24 hours for cases deemed urgent.)

Notifications must be made securely in order not to breach patient confidentiality – telephone, letter, secure fax and encrypted email may be used. The local Health Protection Unit should be contacted for advice. For information on how to contact the local Health Protection Unit go to: http://www.hpa.org.uk/AboutTheHPA/WhoWeAre/ LocalServices/.

The healthcare environment

Table 9 sets out the finishes recommended for the ward environment.

Table 9 Finishes recommended for the ward environment

Room type	Ceiling finish	Floor finish	Wall finish
Patient bed areas Consulting rooms Clean utility room	Any of the following: • Jointless or concealed grid with smooth imperforate finish • Jointed or concealed grid with smooth imperforate finish • Jointed or exposed grid with textured or perforated surface	Seamless flooring or sheet system	Emulsion or heavy-duty emulsion
Dirty utility room Assisted bath/ shower rooms	Any of the following: • Jointless or concealed grid with smooth imperforate finish • Jointed or concealed grid with smooth imperforate finish	Seamless flooring or sheet system or Slip-resistant sheet system	Heavy-duty emulsion or PVC sheet
Toilets	Any of the following: • Jointless concealed grid with smooth finish, resistant to humidity • Jointed exposed grid with smooth finish, resistant to humidity	Slip-resistant seamless flooring or slip-resistant sheet system	Humidity-resistant paint or PVC sheet
Offices Stores Corridors	Jointed or exposed grid with textured or perforated surface Jointed or exposed grid with textured or perforated surface	Seamless flooring or sheet system or textile flooring Seamless flooring or sheet system	Paint Heavy-duty emulsion

Fixtures and fittings

The following standards should be met, with facilities used as described:

HAND WASHING FACILITIES Hand washbasins should be used for hand washing alone and not for any other purpose. The disposal of water used for washing patients, beverages and intravenous fluids, etc., should be done elsewhere as using hand washbasins for disposal can lead to contamination of the sink and ultimately hand contamination and outbreaks of infection.

- Hand washbasins:
  - should be wall mounted, not counter-sunk, as the latter allows water to pool around the edges, which supports bacterial growth;
  - should not have a plug or be capable of taking a plug, as hands should be washed under running, not static, water;
  - should not have an overflow, as this supports bacterial growth and can lead to hand contamination;

- o should be provided in a ratio of one basin for every four beds in new or planned facilities (one per six beds is accepted in older facilities).
- Taps:
  - o should be wall/panel mounted, not countersunk or integral to the hand washbasin, which allows water to pool and supports bacterial growth;
  - o should be sensor/wrist/elbow operated;
  - o should be mixer taps;
  - o must be positioned so that the water does not flow directly into the drainage aperture, as this can lead to splashing.
- Soap dispensers:
  - o should use cartridge refills – refillable dispensers should not be used;
  - o should be wall mounted;
  - o should be close to the hand washbasin.
- Paper towel dispensers:
  - o should be wall mounted;
  - o should be close to the hand washbasin.
- Alcohol handrub:
  - o should be available at the point of care (in a bottle with a pump dispenser attached) on the patient's locker/end of bed or carried by staff in the form of personal bottles (known as 'tottles'); provision of alcohol handrub at the point of care requires risk assessment for areas where there are vulnerable patients, such as the elderly and children;
  - o pump dispenser nozzles should be cleaned regularly to avoid a 'plug' of gel forming, which can lead to the gel squirting into the face/eyes;
  - o bottles should be discarded when empty and not refilled;
  - o pump dispensers should be discarded when the bottle is empty.
- Waste disposal:
  - o there should be a clinical waste bin and a domestic waste bin in each clinical area to support easy waste disposal and correct waste segregation;
  - o a domestic waste bin should be available next to hand washbasins for disposal of paper towels.

LEGIONELLA CONTROL   The maintenance team in your organisation will have a programme for flushing 'low-use outlets' on a weekly basis to reduce the risk of Legionella. A low-use outlet is a tap, shower, toilet or any facility from which water flows that is not used regularly every day.

BEDS   Beds should be spaced with 3.6 metres between their centres. In new and planned builds there should be four beds to a bay.

SEATING   All chairs in hospitals should have impervious, washable coverings in order that they can be cleaned and disinfected.

FLOOR COVERINGS   Flooring should be washable and impervious in clinical areas – there should be no carpeting in clinical areas.

DIRTY UTILITY   The dirty utility should be regarded as a 'dirty' area. It should be used or disposal and there should be a dedicated disposal sink and a sluice hopper or macerator plus a separate hand washbasin to allow staff to clean their hands after waste disposal, commode cleaning, glove removal, etc.

The dirty utility should not be used for storage, other than for commodes. Where space is limited and items are stored there, they should be toilet-related items such as bedpan liners, urinals, vomit bowls and incontinence pads. All items should be stored in their original packaging until required to minimise the risk of contamination from splashing or via contaminated hands.

CLEAN UTILITY   The clean utility should be regarded as a 'clean' area and not used for disposal. There should be a hand washbasin to allow staff to wash their hands before and after preparing medication.

Control of substances hazardous to health (COSHH)

COSHH is the law that requires employers to control substances that are hazardous to health, i.e. substances including chemicals, products containing chemicals, fumes, dusts, vapours, mists, nanotechnology gases and asphyxiating gases and biological agents (germs) that are regarded as toxic, very toxic, harmful, corrosive or irritant.

Some of the substances you use everyday at work, e.g. oxygen, hydrogen peroxide solution, sodium hypochlorite, are regarded as 'hazardous to health' and must be used and stored in accordance with COSHH regulations.

Substances subject to COSHH regulations are marked using 'hazard symbols', which indicate the risk associated with use of that substance.

Hazard symbols

The symbols in Figure 5 indicate that a substance is hazardous to health and must be used and stored in accordance with COSHH regulations.

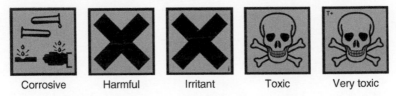

| Corrosive | Harmful | Irritant | Toxic | Very toxic |

Figure 5   Symbols indicating that a substance is hazardous to health

The symbols in Figure 5 are being replaced with new international symbols (shown in Figure 6) but will be visible on items manufactured before 2009, when the new symbols were introduced.

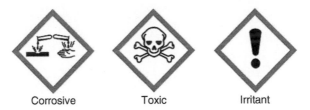

| Corrosive | Toxic | Irritant |

Figure 6   New international symbols

The definitions given above for these symbols is the simplest – each symbol has a broader definition depending on the substance it is applied to.

It is imperative that you follow local guidance in your place of work to ensure that you use and store COSHH substances safely, as failure to do so could result in harm.

Symbols used on medical devices

These are shown in Figure 7.

Temperature limits – both higher and lower limits may be given

Do not use if packaging is damaged

Protect from sunlight

Caution – check for specific warnings or precautions

Batch number or code or lot number

Read the instructions for use

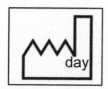

Date of manufacture, will include year, may include month and day

Figure 7 Symbols used on medical devices and their meaning

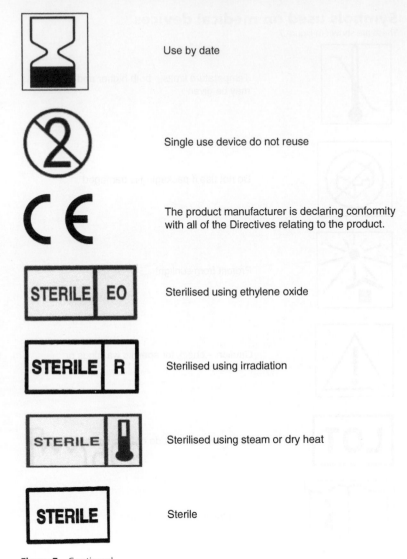

Use by date

Single use device do not reuse

The product manufacturer is declaring conformity with all of the Directives relating to the product.

Sterilised using ethylene oxide

Sterilised using irradiation

Sterilised using steam or dry heat

Sterile

Figure 7 Continued

Antibiotics

This section is broken down into the following subsections: overview, prescribing, administration, side effects and toxicity, penicillin allergy, antibiotic stewardship, classification and resistance

Overview, prescribing, administration, side effects and toxicity, penicillin allergy and antibiotic stewardship

OVERVIEW   Antibiotics are drugs that act against bacteria, either killing them or stopping them from growing and dividing. They are an essential part of modern medicine and at any given time around one-third of hospital inpatients will be on antibiotics. Their role is not only to treat infections but also to prevent them – many procedures and operations would be impossible to perform without antibiotic prophylaxis.

The popularity and widespread use of antibiotics is also their downfall, in that overuse of antibiotics is contributing to problems with resistance. Antibiotics are the only type of medicine where the choice of therapy for one patient can affect diseases suffered in the future by another, by generating antibiotic-resistant organisms that may reach a new host by cross-infection.

PRINCIPLES OF ANTIBIOTIC PRESCRIBING

- Know the likely diagnosis.
- Send cultures before starting antibiotics.
- Antibiotics should only be given when necessary – e.g. draining an abscess may cure it without the need for antibiotics.
- The antibiotic chosen should be active against the likely pathogens while being as narrow spectrum as possible.
- Bactericidal antibiotics are preferred for severe or deep-seated infections and for immunocompromised patients.
- Pharmacokinetics – the antibiotic must achieve adequate levels at the site of infection.
- Keep the duration as short as possible.
- Switch IV to oral as soon as possible, usually by 48 hours.
- Cost – use the cheaper options where possible and bear in mind the cost of administration (greater if multiple doses a day) and of monitoring levels.
- Know the side-effect profile and ensure it is acceptable for your patient.
- Antibiotic prescriptions for inpatients should be reviewed daily.

ROUTES OF ADMINISTRATION OPTIONS INCLUDE:

- Oral (including nasogastric, via PEG or RIG)
- Intravenous (in divided doses or continuous infusion)
- Intramuscular
- Topical
- Rectal
- Rarely, other methods, e.g. nebulised, intra-thecal or intra-vitreal

In most instances, oral administration is preferred where possible.

SIDE EFFECTS AND TOXICITY   Any antibiotic may have side effects; check an up to date *British National Formulary* for further details.

Aminoglycosides such as gentamicin can be toxic to the ear and kidneys at concentrations close to therapeutic. Therefore the dose must be calculated taking into account the patient's weight, renal function and age. Monitoring levels is essential. There are a variety of dosing schedules available: use your hospital's guidelines and liaise with Pharmacy or Microbiology if problems are encountered.

Clostridium difficile infection is acquired when antibiotic use disturbs the normal bowel flora. In theory any antibiotic can cause this, but some antibiotics such as cephalosporins and ciprofloxacin are particularly implicated and are best avoided in high-risk patients such as the over-65s.

PENICILLIN ALLERGY   Approximately 10% of patients report penicillin allergy. It is important to get a detailed history from them or to check with their GP if inadequate details are given. This helps to establish whether the patient can safely be given penicillins or other beta-lactam antibiotics. A 10% cross-reactivity between penicillins and cephalosporins is frequently cited but is thought to be an overestimate.

- Often the reported reaction was not a genuine allergy; nausea, vomiting and diarrhoea are often not true allergies.
- A low-grade allergic reaction such as a flat non-itchy rash would prevent use of penicillins, but it is usually safe to give other beta lactam antibiotics.
- A severe reaction such as facial swelling, urticarial rash, breathlessness or anaphylaxis would usually prevent use of any beta lactam antibiotic if a suitable alternative were available.

All drug allergies should be documented on the drug chart. Seek advice from Microbiology or Pharmacy if required.

ANTIBIOTIC STEWARDSHIP   Antibiotic stewardship requires prudent prescribing, usually based around an antibiotic policy, with an ongoing programme of education, audit, revision and update.

The 'Start Smart – Then Focus' initiative is a useful framework for antibiotic stewardship in secondary care. It is important to be familiar with the principles, as prescribing practice and audits in your organisation are likely to be based on this guidance. The principles for Start Smart are given below:

- Do not start antibiotics in the absence of clinical evidence of bacterial infection.
- If there is evidence/suspicion of bacterial infection, use local guidelines to initiate prompt effective antibiotic treatment.
- Document on drug chart and in medical notes: clinical indication, duration or review date, route and dose.
- Obtain cultures first.
- Prescribe single-dose antibiotics for surgical prophylaxis, where antibiotics have been shown to be effective.

Then Focus is:

- Review the clinical diagnosis and the continuing need for antibiotics by 48 hours and make a clear plan of action – the 'Antimicrobial Prescribing Decision'.
- The five Antimicrobial Prescribing Decision options are:
  1. Stop
  2. Switch IV to oral

3. Change
4. Continue
5. Outpatient parenteral antibiotic therapy (OPAT).

It is essential that the review and subsequent decision is clearly documented in the medical notes.

Classification and resistance

CLASSIFICATION   Antibiotics are classified according to their mechanism of action against bacteria.

Cell wall synthesis inhibitors

These prevent the peptidoglycan component of the cell wall from forming and as a result the bacterial cell dies, i.e. they have a bactericidal action. This group includes:

• Beta-lactams (penicillins, cephalosporins and carbapenems such as meropenem)
• Glycopeptides (such as vancomycin and teicoplanin)

Protein synthesis inhibitors

These inhibit bacterial protein synthesis and thus prevent the bacterial cell from growing and reproducing. Most antibiotics in this group are bacteriostatic (i.e. they stop bacterial growth without killing them) except for the aminoglycosides, which are bactericidal. This group includes:

• Aminoglycosides (such as gentamicin)
• Macrolides (such as erythromycin)
• Tetracyclines (such as doxycycline)
• Chloramphenicol
• Fusidic acid
• Oxazolidinones (linezolid)

Nucleic acid synthesis inhibitors

These prevent bacterial DNA synthesis by a variety of mechanisms:

• Quinolones such as ciprofloxacin are DNA gyrase inhibitors, which prevent DNA supercoiling.
• Antifolate antibiotics such as trimethoprim affect the production of pyrimidine and purine 'building blocks' needed for DNA synthesis.
• Rifamycins such as rifampicin inhibit RNA polymerase.
• Nitroimidazoles such as metronidazole disrupt DNA structure.

RESISTANCE   Resistance is a natural, evolutionary response of bacteria to antibiotic use. Several factors drive the rise of antibiotic resistance, including antibiotic overuse in primary and secondary healthcare and in the farming industry. Poor infection control measures will allow resistant strains to spread. Poor patient compliance (such as not completing the prescribed course of antibiotics) also leads to resistance.

Resistance to antibiotics is becoming a genuine problem in clinical practice. It means that first-line antibiotics are less likely to be effective and that treatment options are limited. Further information is available from the British Society for Antimicrobial Chemotherapy www.bsac.org.uk and Antibiotic Action http://antibiotic-action.com/.

Resistance may be **intrinsic** (when certain bacteria are innately resistant to an antibiotic, usually because it does not possess a target site for the antibiotic or are impermeable to it) or may be **acquired** by one of the following mechanisms:

* Altered target site – changes in the target site may result in lower affinity for the antibiotic or additional target enzymes may emerge that are unaffected by the drug.
* Altered uptake or efflux – effective drug concentration in the bacterial cell can be decreased, either by reduced permeability or by actively pumping the drug back out of the bacterial cell.
* Antibiotic-inactivating enzymes – these occur particularly against beta lactams (beta lactamase/extended spectrum beta lactamase/carbapenemase producers) and aminoglycosides.

4   A–Z of Infections

Acinetobacter

Acinetobacter is a family of Gram-negative bacteria that originate in the environment but which can cause clinical infections, particularly in intensive care or high-dependency patients. Some strains are multiresistant and are known as MRAB (multiresistant *Acinetobacter baumanii*).

SPREAD   Spread is by direct person-to-person contact and indirect contact via contaminated surfaces or medical equipment.

INFECTIOUS PERIOD   This is potentially indefinite, as people who are colonised with MRAB may remain positive for months or years; the risk of transmission can be minimised by using the precautions below. Thorough environmental cleaning is needed if the environment/equipment is contaminated with MRAB, as it can survive for days or weeks in the environment.

INFECTION CONTROL PRECAUTIONS   These are required for MRAB (but not for sensitive strains).

1	Isolation	Required
2	Hand washing	Required
3	Gloves	Required
4	Apron	Required
5	Mask	Not required
6	Eye protection	Not required

STAFF   Staff should follow the precautions above but there are no other requirements.

VISITORS   There are no special precautions/restrictions for visitors.

PATIENT TRANSFER   This should be minimised for patients with MRAB – only essential transfers should be made and the receiving ward/department should be informed in advance.

The environment where the patient is cared for should be cleaned thoroughly after they leave, *before* any other patients are moved into the bed space.

MORE INFORMATION   Infections caused by *Acinetobacter* include urinary tract infections, wound infections, pneumonia and bacteraemia. There are several subtypes of *Acinetobacter* but from an infection control perspective the main issue is whether this is a

Rapid Infection Control Nursing, First Edition. Shona Ross and Sarah Furrows.
© 2014 John Wiley & Sons, Ltd. Published 2014 by John Wiley & Sons, Ltd.

multiresistant *Acinetobacter baumanii* (MRAB) or not. MRAB are so resistant to antibiotics that infections with MRAB can be very difficult to treat; therefore patients known to have MRAB require enhanced infection control precautions to minimise spread. Patients with other forms of *Acinetobacter* generally only require standard principles of infection control. If in doubt, seek advice from a microbiologist or the local Health Protection Unit.

Outbreaks of MRAB may occur. Any outbreak or cluster of infections (i.e. more than one case at one time) should be discussed with the local microbiologist or Infection Control Team and must be reported to the Health Protection Unit.

SCREENING   Screening for MRAB is not usually required. In units with a high number of cases it may be arranged via the local microbiology laboratory – discuss with them before sending swabs. A full screen requires swabs from nose, throat, perineum, rectum and any wounds, including tracheostomy.

Adenovirus

Adenoviruses are a group of viruses that can cause respiratory infections, conjunctivitis, diarrhoea and rashes. These infections are seen more frequently in children than in adults. Infections are usually mild but can be more serious, particularly in the immunosuppressed.

SPREAD BY

* Direct contact with infected persons, primarily via contact with infectious body fluids such as respiratory secretions or by faecal–oral transmission.
* Indirect contact via fomites, e.g. by using towels contaminated with secretions as above.
* Waterborne spread can occur, for example, in poorly chlorinated swimming pools.

INFECTIOUS PERIOD

The incubation period is variable but is typically 4–5 days for respiratory infection and up to 3 weeks for conjunctivitis.

Transmission can occur during the incubation period prior to the onset of symptoms, during the illness, and can sometimes occur after the illness: some patients develop a persistent adenovirus infection of the tonsils, adenoids or intestines and can shed virus for months or years. For practical purposes in most situations, a patient should be regarded as potentially infectious until their symptoms have fully resolved.

INFECTION CONTROL PRECAUTIONS

1	Isolation	Preferred*
2	Hand washing	Required
3	Gloves	Required
4	Apron	Required
5	Mask	Not required
6	Eye protection	Not required unless risk of eye splash

*Isolation is always preferable but may be prioritised as follows: it is essential if the patient has diarrhoea or a rash; if symptoms are respiratory the patient should ideally be isolated but could alternatively be nursed alongside other patients with respiratory symptoms.

STAFF   No additional precautions are required.

VISITORS   Visiting should be restricted to a minimal number of adult visitors during the acute phase of the illness.

PATIENT TRANSFER   This may be permitted but should be kept to a minimum during the acute phase, particularly if the patient has diarrhoea. The receiving ward/department should be informed of the diagnosis prior to moving the patient.

MORE INFORMATION   Outbreaks of adenoviral conjunctivitis may be seen in institutions and should be discussed with the microbiologist and/or Health Protection Unit. Most adenovirus infections are self-limiting. Antivirals are not usually given.

Anthrax

Infection with the bacterium *Bacillus anthracis*. Anthrax is very uncommon and most cases are associated with injecting drug use, imported from overseas, or rarely linked to bioterrorism. Anthrax is a notifiable disease.

SPREAD BY
- Anthrax is not easily spread from person to person.
- Most cases in the UK are seen in people who inject drugs contaminated with anthrax spores.
- Direct contact with skins of infected animals imported from countries where anthrax is more common (e.g. during tanning or other processing) can cause cutaneous or inhalational anthrax.
- Consumption of meat from an infected animal can cause intestinal anthrax.
- Bioterrorism using anthrax spores has occasionally been reported.

INFECTIOUS PERIOD   The incubation period is up to a week. Infected patients are not generally infectious to others, but there is a theoretical risk of transmission via blood and body fluids, so patients are assumed to be infectious for the duration of hospitalisation.

INFECTION CONTROL PRECAUTIONS

1	Isolation	Not required
2	Hand washing	Required
3	Gloves	Required for contact with blood/body fluids
4	Apron	Required for contact with blood/body fluids
5	Mask	Required only for theatre procedures (surgical mask)
6	Eye protection	Required only for procedures where splashing of blood/body fluids may occur

STAFF   No additional precautions are required.

VISITORS   No further restrictions.

PATIENT TRANSFER   Patient transfer should be kept to a minimum and the receiving ward/department must be informed of the diagnosis.

SPECIMENS   The laboratory must be warned in advance of any specimens being sent from patients with possible or confirmed anthrax. Specimens must not be sent via a pneumatic (air tube) transport system.

BLOOD AND BODY FLUID SPILLAGES   Blood and body fluid spillages must be managed wearing gloves and an apron as a minimum, with a mask and eye protection worn if splashing is possible.

A chlorine-releasing agent should be used to disinfect blood and body fluid spillages at a concentration of 10000 parts per million available chlorine. The solution must be allowed 10 minutes of contact tlme with the contaminated surface in order to ensure disinfection.

PATIENT'S CLOTHING   Patient's clothing may potentially carry anthrax spores. If clothing is visibly contaminated with blood or body fluids, it should be discarded as clinical waste (with the patient's permission); if it is contaminated with powder (e.g. their drug supply), discuss with Microbiology; if it appears clean, place it in a sealed plastic bag and allow relatives to take it home for laundering in a separate hot wash.

LINEN   Treat as infected; any linen grossly contaminated with blood or body fluid should be discarded as clinical waste.

MORE INFORMATION   Anthrax is primarily an animal infection and its spores can survive in the environment for prolonged periods. It is rarely seen in the UK.
Anthrax infection may be:

• Cutaneous (skin) anthrax
• Inhalation anthrax
• Injection anthrax – seen in people who inject drugs contaminated with anthrax spores
• Intestinal anthrax

All of these are serious infections that can be fatal.

Campylobacter

Campylobacter is the commonest reported bacterial cause of intestinal infection in England and Wales. Caused by infection with the bacterium *Campylobacter jejuni* or *Campylobacter coli*. Confirmed cases should be reported to the local Health Protection Unit.

SPREAD BY

- Eating undercooked meat (especially poultry) or unpasteurised milk contaminated with *Campylobacter*.
- Contact with infected persons, pets (mainly puppies and kittens) or farm animals (pigs, sheep, rodents and birds may also be sources of infection).
- Many cases are travel associated.

INFECTIOUS PERIOD

- The incubation period is 1 to 11 days (usually 2 to 5 days).
- Typically, cases are infectious from the onset of diarrhoea until 48 hours after their first formed stool.
- In severe or prolonged illness the case can remain infectious for 2 to 7 weeks unless treated with antibiotics.

INFECTION CONTROL PRECAUTIONS

1	**Isolation**	Required
2	**Hand washing**	Required
3	**Gloves**	Required
4	**Apron**	Required
5	**Mask**	Not required
6	**Eye protection**	Not required

Strict adherence to hand washing with soap and water by staff, the patient and visitors is essential. If the patient has a poor hand washing technique they should be assisted to clean their hands properly, particularly after defecating.

STAFF

- Wash hands with soap and water before and after contact with the patient, their belongings and their surroundings.
- Wear gloves for all patient contact, including bed making.
- Wear an apron for all patient contact, including bed making.
- Symptomatic staff should stay off work until 48 hours after their first formed stool.

VISITORS   Visitors must wash their hands with soap and water before and after they visit. They should not eat or drink in the patient's room. Symptomatic visitors should be advised not to visit until 48 hours after their first formed stool.

PATIENT TRANSFER   If transferring the patient between wards/departments, inform the receiving ward/department that the patient has *Campylobacter* and that isolation precautions are required.

MORE INFORMATION   *Campylobacter* is an important cause of diarrhoeal illness in all age groups, causing 5–14% of diarrhoea worldwide.

Immunocompromised persons are at greater risk of infection, likely to have more severe symptoms, more likely to have recurrences and to become chronic carriers.

Cellulitis

This is a soft tissue infection, which is most commonly seen in the legs but can occur at any site.

SPREAD BY   Bacteria may enter the soft tissues via a break in the skin such as an ulcer, wound or insect bite.

Cellulitis is most commonly caused by autoinfection (infection with the patient's own flora) but could be direct person-to-person spread, usually on the hands.

INFECTIOUS PERIOD   Generally up to 24 hours after antibiotic treatment is commenced, but depends on the causative bacterium.

INFECTION CONTROL PRECAUTIONS

1	Isolation	Preferred for the first 24 hours. If not isolated, ensure any wounds are covered
2	Hand washing	Required
3	Gloves	Required for contact with blood/body fluids
4	Apron	Required for contact with blood/body fluids
5	Mask	Required only for procedures where splashing of blood/body fluids may occur
6	Eye protection	Required only for procedures where splashing of blood/body fluids may occur

STAFF   No additional precautions.

VISITORS   No additional precautions.

PATIENT TRANSFER   Patient transfer should be kept to a minimum for the first 24 hours of treatment. Receiving wards/departments must be informed of the diagnosis prior to transfer.

MORE INFORMATION   The commonest causes of cellulitis are *Staphylococcus aureus* or Group A streptococci (GAS). Group C and G streptococci and MRSA are also relatively common causes.

Other bacteria may occasionally cause cellulitis, particularly in diabetics, people with ischaemic legs or the immunocompromised.

Animal bites may be infected by *Pasteurella multocida*, which is important to remember because they need broader spectrum antibiotics.

Chickenpox

Chickenpox is an acute viral illness caused by varicella zoster virus (VZV), a herpes virus.

Chickenpox is best known for its characteristic itchy vesicular rash, which resembles tiny fluid-filled blisters that appear in crops over 3–5 days, mostly on the trunk and face. Many patients also have fever and coryzal (cold-like) symptoms; some have no symptoms other than the rash. Asymptomatic chickenpox does not occur.

SPREAD BY

- Direct person-to-person contact.
- Indirect contact with items recently contaminated with vesicular or mucous membrane secretions.
- Droplet or airborne spread.

In practice, 15 minutes in the same room or bay as an infectious patient, or face-to-face contact for any length of time, is regarded as sufficient to transmit infection. Chickenpox is one of the most contagious infections known, infecting up to 90% of susceptible contacts.

INFECTIOUS PERIOD   The incubation period is 10 to 21 days from exposure, usually 14–16 days. The infectious period is from 2 days before the spots appear until they have crusted over (usually 5–6 days after onset).

INFECTION CONTROL PRECAUTIONS

1	Isolation	Required
2	Hand washing	Required
3	Gloves	Required
4	Apron	Required
5	Mask	Not required
6	Eye protection	Not required

- Isolate the patient in a single room, preferably with negative pressure ventilation.
- Wash hands before and after contact with the patient, their belongings and their surroundings. Alcohol handrub can be used for hand hygiene, providing hands look and feel clean.
- Wear gloves and an apron for all patient contact, including bed making.

STAFF

- All healthcare workers (HCWs) caring for patients with chickenpox must be certain that they have had chickenpox in the past or otherwise should have been vaccinated against VZV. If in doubt contact Occupational Health to arrange to have blood tested for VZV IgG.
- Pregnant HCWs with no immunity or uncertain immunity must avoid contact with chickenpox and have blood taken to determine their immune status.
- HCWs suspected of having chickenpox must report to Occupational Health. All patient contact must stop immediately.
- Any HCW who thinks they may have chickenpox infection must go off sick immediately (report to line manager and Occupational Health) and remain off work for five days after the onset of the rash, or until the lesions have crusted over.
- HCWs should have their immunity to chickenpox tested by Occupational Health at the time of joining the organisation. A vaccine is available for non-immune staff via Occupational Health.

VISITORS   Inform visitors of the infection and only allow those with a past history of/ known immunity to chickenpox to visit.

PATIENT TRANSFER   Only move the patient if absolutely necessary and inform the receiving area of their chickenpox status prior to transfer.

CONTACT TRACING   Patients not immune to chickenpox who have any of the following:

* Face-to-face contact with an infectious patient;
* 15 minutes in the same room as an infectious patient

should have blood tested for varicella antibodies (record 'varicella exposure' and the date of exposure on the lab form) and be isolated/nursed in a bay with others exposed for 10–21 days (the incubation period). Anyone with a history of chickenpox is immune; those without a history should be tested for varicella zoster antibody.

MORE INFORMATION   Persons at risk of severe disease include:

* immunosuppressed patients;
* pregnant women;
* babies whose mothers develop chickenpox between seven days before delivery and seven days after;
* non-immune babies exposed to chickenpox or shingles in the first week of life, or whilst still in intensive care.

People in these groups may be offered varicella zoster immunoglobulin (VZIG) if they have a significant exposure to VZV. Other individuals (adults) who have had significant exposure to VZV but are not eligible to receive VZIG may be offered aciclovir as post-exposure prophylaxis.

Decisions on VZIG or aciclovir prophylaxis should be made after discussion with the Occupational Health and Microbiology departments.

Cholera

This is an acute intestinal infection caused by the bacterium *Vibrio cholerae*. Cholera is a notifiable disease.

SPREAD BY   Consumption of contaminated water or shellfish, or other food washed in contaminated water. Person-to-person transmission is not common. Cholera is an imported (travel-associated) disease in the UK.

INFECTIOUS PERIOD   The incubation period is 1–5 days. Patients are considered infectious until 48 hours after the first normal stool. The organism may still be present in the stool for longer periods, but the risk of transmission from a patient with formed stools is low.

INFECTION CONTROL PRECAUTIONS

1	**Isolation**	Required
2	**Hand washing**	Required
3	**Gloves**	Required
4	**Apron**	Required
5	**Mask**	Not required
6	**Eye protection**	Not required

STAFF NO ADDITIONAL PRECAUTIONS.

VISITORS   Should be kept to a minimum until the patient is stabilised.

PATIENT TRANSFER   Infected patients should be managed on an Infectious Diseases Unit if possible. Other transfers should be kept to a minimum until the diarrhoea has settled. The receiving ward/department should be informed of the diagnosis prior to transfer.

MORE INFORMATION   Cholera presents with sudden onset of profuse, painless, watery diarrhoea sometimes described as 'rice-water stools'. There may be vomiting and leg cramps. Severe cases may lose up to a litre of fluid per hour and rapid fluid replacement is important. Antibiotic use should be guided by sensitivities.

Diagnosis is by stool culture. Ensure the travel history is given with the culture request.

Cholera vaccination is available but plays no part in the management of contacts or the control of outbreaks.

Clostridium difficile

Clostridium difficile is a common and serious cause of diarrhoea in hospital inpatients. It is a spore-forming organism. The spores are dispersed into the environment when an infected person has diarrhoea. At greatest risk of infection are the over-65's, those exposed to spores, e.g. in a healthcare environment, and those on antibiotics.

SPREAD BY   Ingestion of spores via contaminated hands. Hands can become contaminated from contact with an infected person or contaminated equipment/environment. Therefore a high standard of hand hygiene, environmental and equipment cleanliness is essential to minimise the risk of spread. Chlorine-releasing agents at a strength of 1000 parts per million (ppm) should be used daily for disinfection of surfaces.

INFECTIOUS PERIOD   A person is infectious whilst they have diarrhoea. Once the diarrhoea settles, they may still excrete spores in the stool for weeks or months but the spores are less likely to contaminate the environment or be transmitted to other people. Isolation precautions should only be stepped down after discussion with the Infection Prevention and Control Team.

INFECTION CONTROL PRECAUTIONS

1 Isolation	Required
2 Hand washing	Required – use soap and water
3 Gloves	Required
4 Apron	Required
5 Mask	Not required
6 Eye protection	Not required

- Isolate the patient in a single room, preferably within two hours of diagnosis.
- Wash hands before and after contact with the patient, their belongings and their surroundings. Alcohol handrub should not be used for hand hygiene, as it has not been proven to destroy *Clostridium difficile* spores.
- Wear gloves for all patient contact, including bed making.
- Wear an apron for all patient contact, including bed making.

STAFF   Staff are at no particular risk of infection. Hands must be washed with soap and water.

VISITORS   Visitors may choose to wear gloves and an apron but it is not strictly necessary, as they will only have contact with the person they are visiting If worn, visitors should be advised to remove gloves and aprons and to wash their hands with soap and water before leaving the patient's room. Hand washing with soap and water for all patient contacts is essential.

PATIENT TRANSFER   The receiving ward/department should be informed that the patient has *Clostridium difficile* infection and the patient should be seen last on the list if going to another department for investigations.

MORE INFORMATION   In the United Kingdom, a two-stage test for *Clostridium difficile* was implemented in 2012. The two-stage test detects glutamate dehydrogenase (GDH) (an antigen produced in high amounts by both toxin and non-toxin producing strains of *Clostridium difficile*) and *Clostridium difficile* toxin (CDT). Test results should be interpreted as follows:

• GDH positive and CDT positive = *Clostridium difficile* infection likely to be present. Isolate the patient and treat for *Clostridium difficile* infection.
• GDH positive and CDT negative = *Clostridium difficile* is present but not producing toxin. Isolate the patient if they are having diarrhoea and discuss with a microbiologist, as treatment for *Clostridium difficile* infection may be required.
• GDH negative and CDT negative = *Clostridium difficile* infection very unlikely to be present. Isolate the patient if they are having diarrhoea.

Note that if *Clostridium difficile* infection is not present, or is unlikely, there may be another infectious cause of diarrhoea symptoms. All patients with diarrhoea should be isolated until an infectious cause is ruled out. Remember the 'SIGHT' guideline:

S Suspect that a case may be infective when there is no clear alternative cause for diarrhoea.
I   Isolate the patient within 2 hours.
G Gloves and aprons must be used for all contacts with the patient and their environment.
H Hand washing with soap and water should be carried out before and after each contact with the patient and the patient's environment.
T   Test the stool for *C. difficile* by sending a specimen immediately.

Creutzfeldt–Jakob disease (CJD)

Creutzfeldt–Jakob disease (CJD) is a prion disease caused by the build-up of abnormal prion proteins in the brain. CJD is sometimes referred to as a transmissible spongiform encephalopathy (TSE).

From an infection control perspective, the most important issue is identifying CJD patients promptly and ensuring that medical equipment used on them is identified and quarantined if necessary.

When a patient known or suspected to have CJD is scheduled to have a procedure or be admitted to hospital, their planned procedure and history should be discussed in advance with the Infection Prevention and Control Team. Surgical/endoscopic pre-assessments should include questions about history of past blood transfusions and past neurosurgery or posterior eye surgery, which are aimed at identifying patients at higher risk of CJD.

SPREAD   CJD is not spread by person-to-person contact. The following were implicated as methods of spread in the past:

- Consumption of contaminated food products (such as beef during the BSE outbreak of the 1980s).
- Blood transfusion (before safeguards were put in place).
- Medical procedures such as growth hormone use, human dura mater grafts, neurosurgery (before safeguards were put in place).

All of these are unlikely to happen now because appropriate safeguards are in place to prevent such transmission.

INFECTIOUS PERIOD   Indefinite.

INFECTION CONTROL PRECAUTIONS

1	Isolation	Not required
2	Hand washing	Required
3	Gloves	Not required
4	Apron	Not required
5	Mask	Not required
6	Eye protection	Required if risk of splash

1. When taking samples or performing biopsies, use standard principles of infection control and single-use disposable equipment wherever possible.
2. Dispose of sharps should be at the point of use.
3. Inform the Infection Prevention and Control Team and the laboratory when samples are taken.
4. Spillages may be dealt with using standard principles of infection control and a chlorine-releasing agent at 10 000 parts per million available chlorine strength.
5. Dispose of all waste (including cleaning tools, gloves, aprons add masks, etc.) as clinical waste.
6. Patients who have CJD or are at increased risk of CJD are usually last on the list in theatre.
7. Following the procedure, routine cleaning of the theatre with detergent is sufficient, providing blood and body fluid contamination and spillages are disinfected with a chlorine-releasing agent at 10 000 parts per million available chlorine strength.
8. Single-use surgical equipment and instruments should be used where possible.

Reusable instruments must be tracked and traced, and this must be discussed with the Infection Prevention and Control Team to determine whether they can be reused.

STAFF   No additional precautions.

VISITORS   No additional precautions.

PATIENT TRANSFER   No restrictions, but the receiving ward/department must be informed of the diagnosis.

MORE INFORMATION   CJD infection damages the brain tissue, causing characteristic 'spongiform' gaps, which give the brain a sponge-like appearance on microscopy. Patients with CJD suffer gradual deterioration of brain function with a combination of neurological and psychiatric symptoms.

There are four main types of CJD:

- Sporadic or classical CJD is the commonest form.
- Variant CJD is caused by exposure to bovine spongiform encephalopathy (BSE, or 'mad cow disease').
- Iatrogenic CJD is caused by medical procedures with contaminated equipment, e.g. surgical instruments or human-derived growth hormone.
- Familial CJD is genetically inherited.

Cryptosporidiosis

Intestinal infection is with the protozoal parasite *Cryptosporidium parvum*, which causes a watery diarrhoea with abdominal cramps. *Cryptosporidium* infection is notifiable.

SPREAD BY   Cysts are excreted in the stool of infected people or animals and may be transmitted by:

* Water-borne spread: swimming in contaminated swimming pools or drinking contaminated water supplies.
* Person-to-person spread in households and nurseries.
* Contact with infected animals, e.g. farm visits.
* Many cases are linked to foreign travel.
* Rarely, consumption of contaminated food such as unpasteurised milk.

Outbreaks are most common in late summer, probably because people travel and swim more at this time of year.

INFECTIOUS PERIOD   The incubation period is 1–28 days (average 7–10 days). Patients are infectious from the start of symptoms and for many weeks after the symptoms have resolved. They can return to school or work once symptom free for 48 hours. They should not swim while symptomatic or for 2 weeks after symptoms have resolved.

INFECTION CONTROL PRECAUTIONS

1	**Isolation**	Required
2	**Hand washing**	Required
3	**Gloves**	Required
4	**Apron**	Required
5	**Mask**	Not required
6	**Eye protection**	Not required

STAFF   No additional precautions.

VISITORS   No additional precautions.

PATIENT TRANSFER   No additional precautions.

MORE INFORMATION

* Cryptosporidiosis can affect anyone but it most commonly affects children aged between 1 and 5 years.
* Immunosuppressed people, particularly those with HIV, may develop a more severe and prolonged infection.
* Diagnosis is by stool microscopy. Ask the laboratory to look for *Cryptosporidium* if it is suspected, as they need to use special stains.
* There is no specific treatment for cryptosporidiosis. It is usually self-limiting, with symptom resolution within 3–20 days. Fluid replacement is important.
* Cysts of cryptosporidium survive well in the environment, sometimes for many months, and are highly resistant to disinfectants, including chlorine. This explains why swimming pool transmission is a particular problem.

Cytomegalovirus (CMV)

Cytomegalovirus (CMV) infection is a common viral infection that is often asymptomatic but can be associated with symptoms of glandular fever, namely fever, sore throat and lymphadenopathy. More than half of the adult population has had CMV infection at some time.

SPREAD   Transmission occurs through body fluids such as saliva and urine, blood or transplanted organs. The commonest route of transmission is by breast-feeding, which is an integral part of the virus life-cycle. Close household contact or sexual contact are also common ways of transferring infection. Vertical, *intra partum* and perinatal transmission from mother to baby may also occur.

INFECTIOUS PERIOD   The incubation period varies depending on the route of infection but is approximately 2–4 weeks. The infectious period may last for many months after a primary infection.

In general, CMV infection is not easily transmitted within healthcare settings and patient isolation is not usually required.

Babies with congenital CMV can excrete high levels of virus and may remain infectious for 5–6 years. Consideration should be given to restricting pregnant staff from caring for such infants, but if this approach is taken it should be emphasised that excretion of virus in babies and young children is very common. Furthermore, the member of staff will be at most risk of acquiring CMV outside hospital in their home.

INFECTION CONTROL PRECAUTIONS

1	Isolation	Not required
2	Hand washing	Required
3	Gloves	Not required
4	Apron	Not required
5	Mask	Not required
6	Eye protection	Not required

STAFF   Pregnant staff members should ideally not care for patients with active CMV infection, although the risk of infection is very low if standard precautions are followed.

VISITORS   No restrictions, although pregnant women must be advised on the potential risk of CMV infection and instructed to wash hands after the visit.

PATIENT TRANSFER   No restrictions.

MORE INFORMATION   CMV infection in pregnancy can cause severe problems for the developing baby, including deafness, retinopathy and developmental delay. CMV can also cause severe infections in the immunosuppressed, such as retinitis, pneumonia or gastrointestinal infections.

Investigation of CMV infection is not routinely required but the following tests are available: serology (testing a serum sample for CMV IgM and IgG), tissue culture and PCR.

Antiviral treatment is not usually indicated but may be used to treat immunocompromised patients or congenital cases.

Dengue fever

Dengue fever is caused by infection with dengue virus. It is an important cause of fever on return from abroad.

SPREAD   Dengue is transmitted by the bite of an infected female *Aedes* mosquito. It cannot be transmitted from person to person. *Aedes* mosquitoes are not present in the UK and therefore transmission cannot occur in the UK.

INFECTIOUS PERIOD   Not applicable, as person-to-person spread does not occur.

INFECTION CONTROL PRECAUTIONS

1	Isolation	Not required
2	Hand washing	Required
3	Gloves	Not required
4	Apron	Not required
5	Mask	Not required
6	Eye protection	Not required

STAFF   No additional precautions.

VISITORS   No additional precautions.

PATIENT TRANSFER   No restrictions.

MORE INFORMATION   Dengue classically presents as a severe flu-like illness with fever. Avoidance of mosquito bites during travel is the best prophylaxis.
There is no vaccine or antiviral drug for dengue. Treatment is supportive.
Up to date information on dengue is available on the NaTHNaC website www.nathnac.org.

Diarrhoea

Diarrhoea is the passage of three or more loose stools in a 24-hour period. There are many possible causes for diarrhoea, not all of which are infections. Diarrhoea should be presumed to be infectious until an alternative diagnosis is made or negative stool samples are obtained.

SPREAD BY   All diarrhoeal infections can be spread by the faecal–oral route; i.e. the organisms are excreted in the stool, which may contaminate surfaces, and will infect people who ingest the organisms. This can happen surprisingly easily, if people touch contaminated surfaces and then put their hands to their mouth, or eat/drink without washing their hands.

Many diarrhoea-causing organisms survive well on surfaces:

- *Shigella* can survive for up to 20 days on surfaces.
- *Clostridium difficile* forms spores, which survive for a long time and are resistant to alcohol and many disinfectants.
- Norovirus can be excreted in vomit and can aerosolise in an area where someone has vomited, so it spreads very easily with a high attack rate (up to 50% of staff have been affected in some outbreaks).

INFECTIOUS PERIOD   This varies by organism, but in general a person with diarrhoea should be considered to be potentially infectious until they have been free of diarrhoea for 48 hours. Even if organisms are still present in the stool, the risk of transmission is much less once the stools are formed. The main exception is *C. difficile*, where excretion of spores may persist for weeks and may contaminate the environment; therefore ongoing isolation is preferred.

INFECTION CONTROL PRECAUTIONS

1	**Isolation**	Required
2	**Hand washing**	Required. Alcohol gel must not be used as an alternative method
3	**Gloves**	Required
4	**Apron**	Required
5	**Mask**	Not required unless risk of aerosol, e.g. cleaning up vomit from a norovirus case
6	**Eye protection**	Not required

ADDITIONAL MEASURES

- Patients with diarrhoea must be given priority for isolation rooms.
- Patients with diarrhoea should have a stool chart to record type and frequency of bowels motions. The Bristol stool form scale is a useful tool to ensure all staff use the same terminology (types 5, 6 and 7 are diarrhoea).
- A stool sample should be sent to the laboratory for testing.
- Laxatives should be stopped unless constipation with faecal fluid overflow is suspected.
- Supportive measures such as fluid management should be put in place.
- Scrupulous adherence to standard principles of infection control should prevent spread of infection to other patients or staff.
- Eating and drinking on the ward should always be discouraged, but is even more important when there are patients (and/or staff) with diarrhoea on the ward.

STAFF   Any staff with diarrhoea should be advised to inform Occupational Health and not to work until they are symptom free for 48 hours. Any outbreaks of diarrhoea (two or more cases) must be discussed with the Infection Prevention and Control Team.

VISITORS

• Should be warned when there is potentially infectious diarrhoea in the ward and should only visit the affected patient if necessary.
• Should be restricted to a maximum of two adult visitors per patient.
• Should be advised that it is in their own best interests not to eat or drink in the patient area.
• Must be encouraged to wash their hands with soap and water before and after visiting.

If there is an outbreak of diarrhoea on a ward it is advisable to stop all visiting until the outbreak is over. Often visitors may themselves bring diarrhoeal infection on to a ward. People with diarrhoea should not be allowed to visit the wards until they have been symptom free for 48 hours.

PATIENT TRANSFER   Transfers from a ward affected by diarrhoea should be avoided unless absolutely necessary and the receiving ward/area must be informed of the diarrhoea before the transfer takes place. Patients with diarrhoea and asymptomatic patients from a ward affected by an outbreak of diarrhoea should go last on all theatre and treatment lists as far as is practical and safe for the patient.

CLEANING AND DISINFECTION   In areas where patients are having diarrhoea, cleaning and disinfection using detergent and water followed by a chlorine-releasing agent at 1000 parts per million available chlorine strength should take place at least twice a day, with additional cleaning of frequently touched areas such as toilets, toilet flush handles, sinks, taps, door handles, light switches, etc. A thorough terminal clean should be performed after discharge.

MORE INFORMATION   **Diarrhoea starting in a hospital/healthcare facility** may be caused by *Clostridium difficile* or norovirus, or non-infectious causes such as laxative use or constipation with overflow. It is unlikely to be due to food poisoning because most institutions use centrally produced food heated under controlled conditions.

Diarrhoea starting in the community may be caused by a variety of infections including: norovirus, other viral gastroenteritis (cause often not determined), *Clostridium difficile*, *Salmonella*, *Shigella*, *Campylobacter*, *Eschterichia coli* O157, *Giardia* or *Cryptosporidium*.

Traveller's diarrhoea occurs after foreign travel. It is often due to acquisition of a toxin-producing strain of *E. coli*, which may not be possible to diagnose on routine laboratory testing. Other causes include: *Campylobacter*, *Salmonella*, *Shigella*, norovirus, *Giardia*, *Cryptosporidium* or, rarely, amoebic dysentery or cholera.

Dysentery is a term used to describe diarrhoea with blood and mucus, which is usually caused by *Shigella* or *Entamoeba*. For infection control purposes there is no difference in management between diarrhoea and dysentery.

Diphtheria

Diphtheria is a rare disease that predominantly affects the throat but can affect nose, eyes or skin. It is caused by toxin-producing strains of the bacteria *Corynebacterium diphtheria* and *Corynebacterium ulcerans*. The Public Health England must be notified of any suspected or confirmed case of diphtheria.

SPREAD   Direct person-to-person spread via droplets of respiratory secretions (such as sneezing) or indirect spread via contact with articles soiled with discharges from infected people. In general, prolonged close contact (such as household contact) is required for transmission.

INFECTIOUS PERIOD   The incubation period for diphtheria is usually 2 to 5 days.

Patients may harbour the organisms in their throat or nose during the incubation period, during their illness or even for many weeks after the illness if inadequately treated. Therefore the infectious period is potentially weeks or months. All carriers should be prescribed antibiotics to eradicate carriage.

INFECTION CONTROL PROCEDURES

1	Isolation	Required
2	Hand washing	Required
3	Gloves	Required
4	Apron	Required
5	Mask	Required
6	Eye protection	Required if splashing possible

The isolation requirements should stay in place until two sets of cultures (nose and throat swabs, plus skin swabs in cutaneous diphtheria), taken over 24 hours after stopping antibiotics and at least 24 hours apart, are negative for *C. diphtheria/ulcerans*. This means patients would be isolated for most or all of their stay.

STAFF   Staff should have a full vaccination history confirmed and documented by Occupational Health. If this is not available, they should not work with this patient and advice should be sought from Microbiology or the Public Health England as to whether to treat the staff member as a contact of the case.

VISITORS   Visiting should be restricted with the numbers kept to a minimum while the patient is still infectious, although household contacts may be allowed to visit. Visitors should adopt the same infection control precautions as staff. Any close contacts of the case should be offered vaccination, usually via their GP.

PATIENT TRANSFER   This should only occur if essential and the receiving ward/department should be informed of their diagnosis. The patient should wear a mask during transfer if he/she has respiratory symptoms.

MORE INFORMATION   Diphtheria is a vaccine-preventable disease and is more common in countries with poor vaccine uptake, such as Russia, Africa and South Asia. UK cases are rare and are usually imported from other countries.

Patients should be immunised in the convalescent stage of their illness, as natural immunity is not always adequate.

Escherichia coli

Escherichia coli (E. coli) is a bacterium that is part of the normal flora of human beings, found in large quantities in the intestines. E. coli does not generally cause illness in these circumstances. It can cause disease if it gets into the wrong place (e.g. if it spreads from the gut to the bladder it causes a urinary tract infection) or if it is a toxin-producing strain.

Infections caused by E. coli include urinary tract infections, intra-abdominal infections (e.g. following ruptured appendix), biliary sepsis, intestinal infections (traveller's diarrhoea or food poisoning), bloodstream infections (bacteremia), neonatal meningitis and ventilator associated pneumonia.

Most cases require only standard principles of infection control. The exceptions to this are multiresistant strains such as ESBL and toxin-producing strains such as E. coli O157, which require enhanced precautions.

SPREAD BY   Ingestion of contaminated food or water, particularly through foreign travel or consumption of undercooked meat or unpasteurised milk, farm visits or by oro-faecal transmission.

Many E. coli infections are autoinfections, where the patient gets infected by their own flora.

INFECTIOUS PERIOD   Indefinite, as the bacteria may become established in the patient's intestine.

INFECTION CONTROL PRECAUTIONS

1	Isolation	Not required unless the patient has a resistant or toxin-producing strain, or has intestinal infection with diarrhoea or vomiting
2	Hand washing	Required
3	Gloves	Not required unless the patient has a resistant or toxin-producing strain, or has intestinal infection with diarrhoea or vomiting
4	Apron	Not required unless the patient has a resistant or toxin-producing strain, or has intestinal infection with diarrhoea or vomiting
5	Mask	Not required
6	Eye protection	Not required

STAFF   The risk of staff acquiring E. coli from a patient is extremely low provided that standard principles of infection control are followed. Hand hygiene is important to prevent transmission on the hands of staff.

VISITORS   Visitors are at low risk of acquiring E. coli from a patient. If the patient has diarrhoea or vomiting, or is known to have a toxin-producing strain, visitors must be reminded not to have food or drink in the patient area as they could acquire E. coli by ingestion. They should wash their hands before and after a visit.

PATIENT TRANSFER   For most E. coli there is no restriction. For a patient with ESBL or toxin-producing strains, transfer is allowed but the receiving ward/area should be informed of their status prior to the transfer. If the patient has diarrhoea, transfer should be discouraged unless clinically necessary.

MORE INFORMATION   The commonest toxin-producing strains of *E. coli* are a group known as VTEC (vero cytotoxin-producing *E. coli*). The most important VTEC strain in the UK is *E. coli* O157, which has caused outbreaks linked with poor hygiene on farm visits or in butchers' shops.

Most *E. coli* is easily treatable with antibiotics, but some strains produce an enzyme called ESBL, which confers antibiotic resistance (see ESBL producers section for further information).

Extended spectrum beta lactamase (ESBL) producers

Extended spectrum beta lactamase (ESBL) is an enzyme that bacteria can produce to break down antibiotics. ESBL producers are multiple antibiotic resistant and require enhanced infection control precautions.

SPREAD BY Oro-faecal transmission or direct contact with body fluids. Research into transmission and risk factors is ongoing. Antibiotic use is a predisposing factor as it selects for resistant bacteria.

INFECTIOUS PERIOD ESBL carriage tends to occur in the intestine and may continue indefinitely.

INFECTION CONTROL PRECAUTIONS

1	Isolation	Preferable. Local policy in low-risk areas may permit patients to be in a bay or public area provided that good hand hygiene and standard precautions regarding disposal of body fluids, particularly urine and faeces, are complied with
2	Hand washing	Required
3	Gloves	Required for handling blood and body fluids
4	Apron	Required for handling blood and body fluids
5	Mask	No
6	Eye protection	No

ADDITIONAL PRECAUTIONS Early identification of ESBL carriage enables procedures to be put in place. If a patient is admitted with a history of ESBL, or if ESBL is identified in a patient sample, liaise with the Infection Prevention and Control Team immediately.

STAFF No additional precautions.

VISITORS No additional precautions.

PATIENT TRANSFER Not usually restricted, but the receiving ward/area should be informed in advance of their ESBL status. Augmented care units such as ITU or neonatal units may have restrictions in place according to local policy.

MORE INFORMATION Several different types of bacteria can produce ESBL – most commonly *E. coli*, but also other bacteria such as *Klebsiella*, *Enterobacter* and other coliform bacteria.

ESBL producers most commonly cause urinary tract infections but can also cause more serious infections such as septicaemia. ESBL infections are more common in the community than in the healthcare setting. ESBL producers are usually resistant to penicillins, cephalosporins, ciprofloxacin, trimethoprim and sometimes to other antibiotics. They may be sensitive to co-amoxiclav and nitrofurantoin, and are generally sensitive to meropenem. Each ESBL must have laboratory sensitivity tests to determine its resistance pattern.

Screening for ESBLs is not usually necessary in primary or secondary care. If screening is required, e.g. during an outbreak in a tertiary referral unit, this should be discussed first with a microbiologist. Rectal swab or stool samples are the most appropriate samples for screening.

ESBL decolonisation is not practical because the ESBL bacteria are carried in the intestine.

Fleas

SPREAD BY   Direct contact with an infested animal/environment. Fleas will not remain on a human but have the ability to jump on to a person, bite and jump off again.

INFECTIOUS PERIOD   Duration of contact with the infested person/animal/environment until infested clothing is removed and/or the infested animal/environment is treated.

INFECTION CONTROL PRECAUTIONS

1	Isolation	Required until infested clothing has been removed
2	Hand washing	Required
3	Gloves	Required until infested clothing has been removed
4	Apron	Required until infested clothing has been removed
5	Mask	Not required
6	Eye protection	Not required

1. Isolation is not required specifically for prevention of transmission but is preferable in order to maintain privacy and dignity
2. Hand washing is required before and after patient contact and after glove removal.
3. Gloves should be worn when handling infested clothing and bedding. In the home they should be worn for contact with an infested environment/infested animals.
4. An apron should be worn for contact with infested clothing/bedding. In the home an apron should be worn for contact with infested animals.

IMPORTANT POINTS   Removal of infested clothing will remove the fleas from the body. No further treatment is required for the patient other than laundering of the clothing.
• Infested clothing/bedding/linen should be laundered at 60°C.
• In hospital, linen should be sent for laundering in an 'infected linen' bag.

STAFF   Staff are not at risk of catching fleas from a patient after infested clothing/bedding has been removed. In the patient's home it will be possible to catch fleas until any pets and the environment are treated. See important points above.

VISITORS   Visitors are not at risk of catching fleas from a patient after infested clothing/bedding has been removed. In the patient's home the risk will be as stated for staff.

PATIENT TRANSFER   There are no infection risks associated with patient transfer provided their infested clothing was removed and laundered. If the patient will require assistance to rid their home or pet(s) of fleas this should be communicated to ongoing care agencies and the local authority if necessary to ensure the required level of support is provided.

MORE INFORMATION   The following additional measures should be implemented ideally before the patient is discharged home:

• In the patient's home environment the carpets should be vacuumed and it may be necessary to treat them with sprays/powders. Pets should be treated for fleas.
• The local authority should be contacted for advice on deinfestation of the home if the infestation is severe or the patient requires assistance.
• It is essential to consult a vet for advice on deinfestation of pets, their bedding and the home environment to avoid harm.

Giardia

Intestinal infection with the protozoan parasite *Giardia lamblia* (also known as *Giardia intestinalis* or *Giardia duodenalis*). *Giardia* infection is a notifiable disease.

SPREAD BY Direct person-to-person contact, particularly if there is poor hygiene, e.g. in a nursery; spread within households is common; consumption of contaminated water or food; swimming in contaminated water.

Many cases are travel-associated, but *Giardia* is fairly common in the UK.

INFECTIOUS PERIOD The incubation period is 5 to 25 days. Patients remain infectious while untreated or if there is treatment failure (approximately 10% of cases).

INFECTION CONTROL PRECAUTIONS

1	**Isolation**	Required
2	**Hand washing**	Required
3	**Gloves**	Required
4	**Apron**	Required
5	**Mask**	Not required
6	**Eye protection**	Not required

STAFF No additional precautions.

VISITORS Advise visitors not to eat or drink in the room and to wash their hands after the visit.

PATIENT TRANSFER The receiving ward/department should be informed of the diagnosis.

MORE INFORMATION Symptoms include diarrhoea (bulky, pale stools – no blood), loss of appetite, nausea and abdominal bloating. Some patients are asymptomatic.

Giardia infection may become chronic and cause ongoing steatorrhoea and malabsorption. Persistent symptoms are sometimes due to lactose intolerance rather than ongoing infection.

Diagnosis is by stool microscopy.

Treatment is with metronidazole. Household members should be screened for infection and treated if positive.

Glandular fever (infectious mononucleosis)

Glandular fever is a common illness caused by acute infection with the Epstein–Barr virus (EBV). It can occur at any age but is seen most commonly in children and young adults. Symptoms include fever, lymphadenopathy and a sore throat. Patients often develop a biochemical hepatitis and an enlarged spleen, which return to normal over time.

SPREAD BY   Close direct contact with an infected person. Transmission requires contact with the saliva of an infected person so requires kissing/sexual contact. Because it is not spread by casual contact and because 90–95% of adults are immune, isolation is not required.

INFECTIOUS PERIOD   The incubation period for glandular fever is 4–6 weeks. The illness may last for up to 2 weeks, with fatigue lasting longer. EBV virus remains latent in a person after the initial infection and may intermittently reactivate, thus becoming potentially transmissible again.

INFECTION CONTROL PRECAUTIONS

1	Isolation	Not required
2	Hand washing	Required
3	Gloves	Not required
4	Apron	Not required
5	Mask	Not required
6	Eye protection	Not required

STAFF   No additional precautions.

VISITORS   Not restricted.

PATIENT TRANSFER   Not restricted.

MORE INFORMATION   Patients with suspected or confirmed glandular fever should never be given amoxicillin, as it can cause a widespread rash if given during glandular fever. Other penicillins, such as penicillin V, are safe to use.

Patients with glandular fever are at risk of splenic rupture and should be advised to avoid contact sports and heavy lifting for at least 1 month after the illness.

Most cases are self-limiting and no specific treatment is required.

The diagnosis may be confirmed by blood tests, either Monospot (EDTA blood to Haematology) or EBV serology (serum via Microbiology/Virology).

Glycopeptide-resistant enterococci (GRE)

This is also known as vancomycin-resistant enterococci (VRE). GRE may colonise or infect patients who have had prolonged hospital stay with antibiotic use, particularly in high-dependency units.

SPREAD BY   GRE are excreted in the stool and are also found in body fluids or on the skin of colonised patients. It survives well in the environment, particularly if the environment is cluttered and dusty.

Direct transfer of GRE may occur from patient to patient on the hands of staff. Indirect transfer of GRE can occur if the environment contains GRE that goes on to the hands of staff or on to equipment.

Outbreaks of GRE infection can occur if hand hygiene or environmental cleanliness are inadequate. This is more likely to happen in high-dependency areas such as ITU/HDU, where there are frequent staff/patient contacts.

INFECTIOUS PERIOD   The infectious period is indefinite as GRE is carried in the intestine and rectum, and therefore decolonisation is impractical.

Rectal swab or stool sample can be used to assess GRE carriage status. However, excretion in the stool can be intermittent, so a single negative in a known colonised patient is not considered sufficient evidence to declare them negative.

Screening for GRE status is not a routine investigation and should be discussed with a microbiologist or infection control nurse.

INFECTION CONTROL PRECAUTIONS

1	**Isolation**	Required
2	**Hand washing**	Required
3	**Gloves**	Required
4	**Apron**	Required
5	**Mask**	Not required unless risk of splash
6	**Eye protection**	Not required unless risk of splash

- Good hand hygiene is paramount in preventing the spread of GRE.
- Known GRE positive patients should be isolated as soon as they are admitted to hospital. Not all hospitals have alerting systems for GRE positive status, so past records should be checked.
- GRE is resistant to many common antibiotics and antibiotic use can actively select for GRE. In general, antibiotics should be avoided where possible in patients with GRE. If antibiotics are genuinely required, discuss with a microbiologist to ensure that the choice is appropriate.

STAFF   No additional precautions.

VISITORS   No restrictions.

PATIENT TRANSFER   This should be restricted to essential transfers only. The receiving ward/department should be informed of the GRE status and the patient should go last on the list if having a procedure.

GRE IN THE COMMUNITY   Many GRE patients will be discharged from hospital to an intermediate care facility or nursing home. At this stage it becomes impractical to continue full isolation precautions, particularly as the GRE is unlikely to cause serious illness in contacts. The decision to step down isolation precautions is ultimately the responsibility of the receiving facility but would generally be justified. Patients who go home do not have to take any special precautions.

MORE INFORMATION   Enterococci are bacteria that are usually found as normal flora in the bowel. They are a common cause of urinary tract infection and may also cause intra-abdominal infection (e.g. after intestinal perforation), wound infection, line infection and endocarditis. They are generally low-grade pathogens that cause only mild infections. Most enterococci are not of infection control significance.

GRE are enterococci that have acquired resistance to glycopeptides (a class of antibiotics that includes vancomycin and teicoplanin). Enhanced infection control precautions are necessary to prevent the spread of resistance. GRE cause the same spectrum of disease as other enterococci (above) and often cause few or no symptoms of infection. If a patient has GRE without clinical infection they are said to be colonised.

Group A streptococcus (GAS)

This bacterium is carried in the nose and/or throat of approximately 10% of the population. It can cause sore throats and skin and soft tissue infections such as cellulitis, impetigo and necrotising fasciitis. Invasive Group A streptococcal infection (iGAS) is notifiable.

SPREAD BY   Direct person-to-person contact on hands or by respiratory secretions.
Airborne spread can occur over short distances, by airborne dispersal from septic lesions or nose/throat carriage. Occasionally indirect spread can occur, e.g. transfer from one patient to another via a dirty laryngoscope handle.
Autoinfections can occur (where a GAS carrier goes on to develop an infection).

INFECTIOUS PERIOD   A patient with GAS infection is infectious from the onset of symptoms until 24 hours after commencing appropriate antibiotics.
A patient or staff member who carries GAS in their throat may be infectious indefinitely. Staff should be treated with antibiotics if they have direct patient contact, particularly contact with wounds.

INFECTION CONTROL PRECAUTIONS

1	**Isolation**	Required until 24 hours of appropriate antibiotic therapy completed
2	**Hand washing**	Required
3	**Gloves**	Required for contact with blood/body fluids
4	**Apron**	Required for contact with blood/body fluids
5	**Mask**	Required only for procedures where splashing of blood/body fluids may occur
6	**Eye protection**	Required only for procedures where splashing of blood/body fluids may occur

STAFF   Staff with severe sore throats should arrange review by Occupational Health or their GP.

VISITORS   Visitor numbers should be restricted for the first 24 hours of treatment. Ask them for details of household contacts to assist the Health Protection Team with their management.
Visitors with severe sore throats should arrange a review by their GP.

PATIENT TRANSFER   Patient transfer should be kept to a minimum for the first 24 hours of treatment. Receiving wards/departments must be informed of the diagnosis.

MORE INFORMATION   Cases of invasive Group A streptococcus (iGAS), i.e. where GAS is cultured from a normally sterile site such as blood, must be reported to the Health Protection Unit, who will arrange further investigations and prophylactic antibiotics for contacts. Seek advice from your local microbiologist.
Two or more cases of GAS infection in a healthcare setting may constitute an outbreak and must be discussed with the Health Protection Unit and a microbiologist.

Group B streptococcus (GBS)

This is also known as *Streptococcus agalactiae*.

SPREAD BY   Infants can pick up the infection from their mother *in utero* during pregnancy or during delivery. In early onset disease (within the first week of life) the source of infection is usually the mother's genital flora. In late onset disease (between the seventh and 90th day of life) it is thought that the infection is acquired, e.g. due to cross-infection. Poor hand hygiene and inadequate cleaning of the environment and equipment are possible methods of spread.

In adults the mechanism of spread is unclear. It is possible that infection may be due to autoinfection (where bacteria in one part of the body are transferred to another part, by the carrier, causing an infection).

INFECTIOUS PERIOD   GBS can be spread for the duration of the time that a person is infected or colonised.

INFECTION CONTROL PRECAUTIONS

1	Isolation	Required for infants
		Not required for adults
2	Hand washing	Required
3	Gloves	Required
4	Apron	Required
5	Mask	Not required
6	Eye protection	Not required

STAFF   Staff are not at particular risk of infection.

VISITORS   The same precautions as for staff should be adopted.

PATIENT TRANSFER   No specific infection control precautions are required for transfer. Inform the receiving area of the patient's GBS infection – infants will require isolation in the receiving ward/department.

MORE INFORMATION   GBS can be found in the gastrointestinal tract and on the skin of men and women and are also part of the normal bacterial flora of the female genital tract. Up to 30% of pregnant women are colonised with GBS in the vagina and/or rectum. GBS infections can occur in men and women of all ages but are most common in infants.

Infant GBS infection

In infants GBS causes meningitis, septicaemia and pneumonia.

Adult GBS infection

In adults, GBS mainly cause urinary tract infections or infection of pre-existing wounds such as diabetic foot ulcers or pressure sores. Less commonly GBS may cause bacteraemia, pneumonia or endocarditis in patients who are elderly or have other underlying problems such as diabetes or malignancy.

Group C and Group G streptococci

Group C streptococcus (*Streptococcus dysgalactiae*) and Group G streptococcus (*Streptococcus canis*) closely resemble Group A streptococcus and cause most of the same diseases, mainly sore throats and skin and soft tissue infections, also eye and ear infections. They occasionally cause septicaemia and endocarditis.

They usually cause milder infections than Group A streptococcus and do not have Public Health implications.

SPREAD BY   Direct person-to-person contact on hands or by respiratory secretions. Airborne spread can occur over short distances, by airborne dispersal from septic lesions or nose/throat carriage.

INFECTIOUS PERIOD   From onset of symptoms until 24 hours after commencing appropriate antibiotics.

INFECTION CONTROL PRECAUTIONS

1	Isolation	Not required
2	Hand washing	Required
3	Gloves	Required for contact with blood/ body fluids
4	Apron	Required for contact with blood/ body fluids
5	Mask	Not required
6	Eye protection	Not required

STAFF   No additional precautions.

VISITORS   No further restrictions.

PATIENTS   No further restrictions.

MORE INFORMATION   Group C streptococci are also animal pathogens. Group G streptococcal infections are often associated with underlying malignancy.

Haemophilus influenzae type B (Hib)

Haemophilus influenzae type B (Hib) is a bacterium present in the nasopharynx that can disseminate to cause severe life-threatening disease. Invasive Hib infection (clinical infection, plus Hib isolated from a normally sterile site) is a notifiable disease in England and Wales.

SPREAD BY   The bacteria live in the nose and throat and are present in nose and throat secretions. They are spread during coughing and sneezing (droplet spread) and by direct contact with these body fluids.

INFECTIOUS PERIOD   Confirmed cases are infectious until 48 hours after antibiotic treatment has started.

INFECTION CONTROL PRECAUTIONSNFECTION CONTROL PRECAUTIONS

1	**Isolation**	Required
2	**Hand washing**	Required
3	**Gloves**	Required
4	**Apron**	Required
5	**Mask**	Required
6	**Eye protection**	Required if there is a risk of splashing to the face

STAFF   Staff are at no particular risk of infection.

VISITORS   Should adopt the same precautions as staff.

PATIENT TRANSFER   Should be avoided during the infectious period. If transfer is necessary the patient should wear a surgical mask to contain coughs and sneezes. The receiving ward/department should be informed of the patient's status prior to transfer.

MORE INFORMATION   *Haemophilus influenzae* type B (Hib) infection can occur at any age but predominantly affects children under five years of age, causing meningitis, pneumonia, epiglottitis, facial cellulitis, bone and joint infections and bacteraemia. It can be fatal; 4–5% of cases die (the rate is higher in infants) and up to 30% of survivors are left with permanent neurological damage, such as mental impairment, convulsions and deafness.

Hib is vaccine-preventable. Since the Hib conjugate vaccine was introduced into the routine childhood immunisation programme in the UK, the incidence of invasive Hib disease has fallen by over 90% across all age groups.

Hand, foot and mouth disease

Hand, foot and mouth disease is a common viral illness caused by infection with Coxsackie virus, a type of enterovirus.

SPREAD BY   Direct contact with faeces (oro-faecal transmission), nasal/pharyngeal secretions or respiratory droplets. Spread can therefore be reduced by hand hygiene and respiratory hygiene.

INFECTIOUS PERIOD   The incubation period is 3–5 days. A person is infectious during the acute illness and for several weeks afterwards, as viral excretion in the stool can persist.

INFECTON CONTROL PRECAUTIONS

1	Isolation	Not usually required, though may be advisable if diarrhoea or significant coryzal symptoms are present
2	Hand washing	Required
3	Gloves	Not required
4	Apron	Not required
5	Mask	Not required
6	Eye protection	Not required

STAFF   No restrictions, though pregnant staff may prefer to avoid contact.

VISITORS   No restrictions, though pregnant visitors may prefer to avoid contact.

PATIENT TRANSFER   No restrictions, but the receiving unit should be informed of the diagnosis.

MORE INFORMATION   Symptoms are generally mild and include fever, a maculopapular or vesicular rash on the hands and feet, and a pharyngitis with vesicles that burst to leave painful ulcers in the mouth. Most cases resolve within 7–10 days.

A single case does not need to be notified, but clusters of cases should be reported to the Health Protection Unit.

Epidemics occur every 2–3 years, with most cases occurring in young children and in the months of July to December.

Laboratory confirmation is not usually necessary but can be performed by viral culture/PCR of stool or viral throat swab; serological testing is of use only in making a retrospective diagnosis.

Hand, foot and mouth disease is not related to the foot and mouth disease that affects cows, sheep and pigs.

There are occasional reports of miscarriage in pregnant women with hand, foot and mouth, but there is no firm evidence of a link.

Hepatitis A virus

Hepatitis A is an acute viral hepatitis caused by infection with the hepatitis A virus. It is a notifiable disease.

SPREAD BY

- Direct person-to-person spread, including sexual transmission.
- Faecal-oral spread (consumption of food/water contaminated with faeces of an infected person).
- Spread via blood (injecting drug use; spread via transfusion of blood products from infected donors has been reported but is rare).

Hepatitis A transmission in the community can be prevented by good hygiene (hand washing after toilet use and before food preparation) and by vaccination of high-risk groups.

IINFECTIOUS PERIOD   The incubation period is around 28 days (range is 15–50 days).
The infectious period is from two weeks before the onset of symptoms until one week after. Some people, particularly children and infants, remain infectious for a week longer. Hepatitis A does not have a chronic carrier state.

INFECTION CONTROL PRECAUTIONS

1	Isolation	Required until one week after the onset of jaundice, or if no jaundice is present, until ten days after onset of symptoms. In infants and children this will be prolonged
2	Hand washing	Required
3	Gloves	Required
4	Apron	Required
5	Mask	Not required
6	Eye protection	Not required

STAFF   Staff should be actively immunised as soon as possible after exposure, but no later than two weeks after exposure. Contact Occupational Health for advice.

VISITORS   Visitors should adopt the same precautions as those advised for staff. Visitors should contact their GP for advice on immunisation, which is advisable for all close personal contacts, including household, sexual and those using illicit drugs.

OTHER PATIENTS   Other inpatients in close contact with a person infected with hepatitis A should be offered immunisation.

PATIENT TRANSFER   If transfer is required inform the receiving area of the patient's hepatitis A status prior to transfer.

MORE INFORMATION   Hepatitis A infection ranges from mild or asymptomatic infection to nausea, vomiting, malaise, hepatitis (liver inflammation with jaundice) and even liver failure. Asymptomatic infection is common in children, but in adults 70–95% of infections cause clinical illness.
Infection is followed by lifelong immunity.

Hepatitis B virus

Hepatitis B is a bloodborne viral infection of the liver caused by infection with the hepatitis B virus. It causes acute hepatitis and may cause long-term liver damage. Hepatitis B is a notifiable disease.

SPREAD BY   Hepatitis B infection is transmitted by direct contact with infected blood or body fluids. Body fluids that may contain hepatitis B virus include: blood/blood products/saliva/cerebrospinal fluid/peritoneal fluid/pleural fluid/pericardial fluid/synovial fluid/amniotic fluid/semen/vaginal secretions/any other body fluid containing blood/unfixed tissues and organs.

Infection can occur if these fluids enter the body via the intravenous/intramuscular/subcutaneous/intradermal/mucosal routes.

Examples of routes of transmission include:

- Use of contaminated/shared equipment during injecting drug use.
- Vertical transmission (mother to baby).
- Sexual transmission.
- Sharps injury.
- Tattooing or body piercing using contaminated equipment.
- Transfusion of infected blood or blood products (this should not happen where screening of blood products is in place).

INFECTIOUS PERIOD   The incubation period ranges from 40 to160 days.

All persons who are Hepatitis B surface antigen (HBsAg) positive are potentially infectious, are likely to have been infectious for a few weeks before the onset of their first clinical symptoms and remain infectious throughout the acute clinical course of the disease and sometimes for longer (carrier state). Blood tests for hepatitis B markers and/or PCR will give further information on infectivity and guide further management.

INFECTION CONTROL PRECAUTIONS

1	Isolation	Not required
2	Hand washing	Required
3	Gloves	Required when blood/body fluid contact is possible
4	Apron	Required when blood/body fluid contact is possible
5	Mask	Required when splashing of body fluids is possible
6	Eye protection	Required when splashing of body fluids is possible
7	Disinfection of blood/body fluid spillages	Chlorine-releasing agents at a concentration of 10 000 parts per million (ppm) available chlorine should be used to disinfect blood/body fluid spillages
8	Waste management	Treat waste as 'clinical waste' and dispose of via clinical waste stream (orange waste sack)
9	Linen and laundry	Items contaminated with blood/body fluids should be treated as 'infectious linen' and bagged accordingly

STAFF   All healthcare workers should be vaccinated against hepatitis B.

If any intravenous/intramuscular/subcutaneous/intradermal or mucosal contact with blood/blood products or any of the body fluids listed above occurs you must attend Occupational Health for risk assessment as a matter of urgency. Hepatitis B vaccine or immunoglobulin may be given if necessary, and this is best done within 24 hours of the event.

VISITORS   No special precautions unless patients are actively bleeding/leaking any of the fluids listed above, in which case gloves and aprons should be worn.

PATIENT TRANSFER   The receiving department/ward must be notified of the patient's hepatitis B status.

MORE INFORMATION   Hepatitis B infection may be asymptomatic or may present with a flu-like illness, nausea and vomiting, sore throat, tiredness and loss of appetite, abdominal discomfort and jaundice.

Hepatitis B is common in Asia, Africa, the Middle East and southern Europe. In the United Kingdom the prevalence of chronic hepatitis B infection is estimated at 0.3%.Hepatitis B is stable on environmental surfaces for at least seven days and it is possible to pick up the virus from inanimate objects.

Those at greatest risk of infection are sexual and close household contacts of an infected person, babies born to hepatitis B mothers, injecting drug users sharing equipment with hepatitis B infected persons and healthcare workers caring for hepatitis B infected patients.

Hepatitis C virus

Hepatitis C is a bloodborne viral infection of the liver caused by infection with the hepatitis C virus (HCV). It causes acute hepatitis and may cause long-term liver damage. Hepatitis C is a notifiable disease.

SPREAD BY

- Direct contact – entry into the bloodstream of hepatitis C infected blood via intravenous access. Examples: injecting drug use; tattooing/body piercing if equipment is contaminated; blood/blood product transfusion if blood not screened for infection. Sharing razors or toothbrushes can also spread infection.
- Perinatal transmission from mother to child also occurs (transmission risk estimated at 5%).
- Sexual transmission is rare but can occur, especially among men who have sex with men. Heterosexual hepatitis C carriers are not routinely advised to use condoms with sexual partners.

INFECTIOUS PERIOD   Indefinite. Blood tests (PCR) can establish whether a person has cleared the infection or is still infectious. If PCR results are not available, treat the patient as potentially infectious.

INFECTION CONTROL PRECAUTIONS

1	**Isolation**	Required only if actively bleeding; otherwise not required
2	**Hand washing**	Required
3	**Gloves**	Required for contact with blood/body fluids
4	**Apron**	Required for contact with blood/body fluids
5	**Mask**	Required only for procedures where splashing of blood/body fluids may occur
6	**Eye protection**	Required only for procedures where splashing of blood/body fluids may occur

1. Persons infected with/carriers of hepatitis C virus need not be isolated unless they are actively bleeding, in which case they should be nursed in a single room.
2. Wash hands before and after contact with the patient, their belongings and their surroundings. Alcohol handrub can be used for hand hygiene providing hands look and feel clean.
3. Wear gloves for contact with blood/body fluids.
4. Wear an apron for contact with blood/body fluids.
5. Wear a surgical facemask if blood/body fluids splashes to the face are anticipated.
6. Wear eye protection if blood/body fluids splashes to the face are anticipated.

STAFF

- In the event of a sharps injury wash the affected area with warm water and soap. Do not squeeze, suck or scrub the area. Cover with a dressing and attend Occupational Health or the Emergency Department. Complete an incident report.
- In the event of a splash injury rinse the affected area with copious amounts of water. If the splash injury was to the mouth do not swallow the water used to rinse out the mouth. Attend Occupational Health or the Emergency Department. Complete an incident report.

VISITORS   Visitors should adopt the same precautions as those advised for staff when the patient is actively bleeding.

PATIENT TRANSFER   If transfer is required inform the receiving area of the patient's Hepatitis C status prior to transfer.

MORE INFORMATION   Hepatitis C infection may be asymptomatic or may present with a flu-like illness, nausea and vomiting, sore throat, tiredness and loss of appetite, abdominal discomfort and jaundice.

Around 15–20% of people infected with hepatitis C will clear their infection within 6 months; the remainder develop a chronic infection that may last for decades. Antiviral treatment for hepatitis C is now available.

Hepatitis C is common worldwide. The United Kingdom is not a high-prevalence country but there are an estimated 216 000 individuals with chronic hepatitis C infection.

Hepatitis D virus

This is also known as HDV, hepatitis delta virus or delta associated hepatitis. Hepatitis D is a virus that causes hepatitis only in the presence of hepatitis B virus. The clinical significance of hepatitis D is that its presence results in more severe disease than infection with hepatitis B alone. From an infection control perspective, hepatitis D virus infection is always associated with a hepatitis B virus infection; therefore the risk of transmission of hepatitis B infection is also present in a patient with hepatitis D virus infection. Hepatitis D infection is notifiable.

SPREAD BY   Entry into the bloodstream of blood or serous body fluids infected with hepatitis D virus via contaminated needles and syringes, plasma derivatives and via sexual intercourse.

INFECTIOUS PERIOD   Patients with hepatitis D virus infection are infectious through-out all phases of the acute infection and probably most infectious just prior to the onset of acute illness.

INFECTION CONTROL PRECAUTIONS

1	Isolation	Not required
2	Hand washing	Required
3	Gloves	Required when blood/body fluid contact is possible
4	Apron	Required when blood/body fluid contact is possible
5	Mask	Required when splashing of body fluids is possible
6	Eye protection	Required when splashing of body fluids is possible

STAFF   If any intravenous/intramuscular/subcutaneous/intradermal or mucosal contact with blood/blood products or any of the body fluids listed above occurs you must attend Occupational Health for risk assessment as a matter of urgency. Hepatitis B vaccine or immunoglobulin may be given if necessary, and this is best done within 24 hours of the event.

VISITORS   No special precautions unless patients are actively bleeding/leaking any of the fluids listed above, in which case gloves and aprons should be worn.

PATIENT TRANSFER   The receiving department/ward must be notified of the patient's hepatitis D virus infection status.

MORE INFORMATION   Hepatitis D can infect patients who already have hepatitis B (superinfection), or a patient could acquire both hepatitis B and D simultaneously (coinfection).

Hepatitis D is uncommon in the United Kingdom and most developed countries.

Risk groups include patients with bleeding disorders, injecting drug users, people who frequently come into contact with blood, those in institutions for the developmentally disabled and, to a lesser extent, men who have sex with men. In the United Kingdom the majority of cases are in people who inject drugs.

Hepatitis B vaccination and reducing sexual activity and needle sharing are the most effective ways to reduce transmission of hepatitis D virus.

Hepatitis E virus (HEV)

Hepatitis E virus is an RNA virus that infects the liver to cause hepatitis. Transmission and clinical features resemble hepatitis A. Hepatitis E infection is a notifiable disease.

SPREAD BY

- Faecal-oral route: Consumption of drinking water or food contaminated with faeces.
- Spread from person to person is rare and occurs in only 1–2% of cases.
- Zoonotic transmission (from animals) has been reported, through consumption of under-cooked pork, deer meat or shellfish.

INFECTIOUS PERIOD   The incubation period is 15–60 days (average 40 days). The patient is infectious before they develop symptoms of infection and remain infectious for up to 14 days after clinical symptoms appear. Immunocompromised patients may remain infectious for longer.

INFECTION CONTROL PRECAUTIONS

1	Isolation	Not required
2	Hand washing	Required
3	Gloves	Required
4	Apron	Required
5	Mask	Not required
6	Eye protection	Not required

STAFF   There are no special precautions although women in the third trimester of pregnancy should not care for the patient until 14 days after the onset of symptoms.

VISITORS   No special precautions although women in the third trimester of pregnancy should not visit the patient until 14 days after the onset of symptoms.

PATIENT TRANSFER   There are no special precautions other than hand hygiene. Communication of the patient's infection status to the receiving department/ward is essential.

MORE INFORMATION   Symptoms of hepatitis E include anorexia, nausea, vomiting, fever, abdominal pain or tenderness and jaundice. It is usually a mild disease but can be severe or fatal in the third trimester of pregnancy (20% mortality in this group), immuno-compromised patients or in those with pre-existing chronic liver disease. Infection does not usually lead to chronic hepatitis or a carrier state.

Hepatitis E is commoner in regions of the world where sanitation and food hygiene are poor (outbreaks have commonly occurred in Asia, Africa and Central America) but transmissions of hepatitis E have occurred in North America, Europe and the United Kingdom.

Hepatitis E is diagnosed by serological testing; discuss with your Microbiology/Virology laboratory.

It is not known whether infection with hepatitis E virus confers lifelong immunity. There is a vaccine for hepatitis E, but it is not yet widely used.

Herpes simplex virus

There are two types of Herpes simplex virus (HSV): Herpes simplex virus 1 (HSV 1) and Herpes simplex virus 2 (HSV 2).

SPREAD BY   HSV is spread by direct contact with saliva during kissing, sexual exposure and contact sports, e.g. scrum pox on the faces of rugby players. It is highly infectious and can easily be transmitted via contaminated hands after touching a lesion.

INFECTIOUS PERIOD   The first time a person has the infection their saliva contains the virus for between 1 and 8 weeks; thus they are infectious throughout that time. In subsequent infections (recurrences) the person will be infectious for about 3 days whilst lesions are moist, until they crust over.

INFECTION CONTROL PRECAUTIONS

1	Isolation	Not required unless infection is extensive
2	Hand washing	Required
3	Gloves	Required for direct patient contact
4	Apron	Required for direct patient contact
5	Mask	Not required
6	Eye protection	Not required

STAFF   Staff with HSV infection should not come into contact with pregnant or postnatal women, infants, burns patients and those with impaired immunity or eczema.

VISITORS   The same precautions as for staff are advisable.

PATIENT TRANSFER   The receiving ward/department should be informed of the patient's HSV infection status. No specific precautions are required for transfer other than hand hygiene after direct patient contact.

MORE INFORMATION   HSV has a pattern of localised primary infection followed by latency and recurrence. HSV 1 typically causes infection of the mouth and gums that leads to swelling and ulceration while HSV 2 is more commonly associated with genital infection; although both can affect the genital tract HSV 2 can rarely cause infection in the mouth. HSV 1 is now responsible for approximately 30% of genital infection as more adolescents enter sexual debut susceptible to both viruses. Asymptomatic/subclinical infection is common.

Other sites such as the eyes and fingers (herpetic whitlow) can become infected through autoinoculation during the primary infection. This is possible because the person touches the infected area and then another area, causing infection, before sufficient antibody has developed to prevent it.

Complications of HSV infection are eczema herpeticum, Bell's palsy, encephalitis, meningitis (both primary and recurrent), erythema multiforme and ocular herpes, which can lead to corneal ulceration and is an ophthalmic emergency.

The diagnosis of HSV may be confirmed by taking a viral swab of the lesion for herpes PCR or cell culture. Serology is difficult to interpret and should not be sent without prior agreement from the laboratory.

Human immunodeficiency virus (HIV)

There are two types of HIV infection: HIV-1 and HIV-2. The latter is endemic in western Africa and is a much more benign infection with a better prognosis compared with HIV-1.

SPREAD BY　Entry of HIV infected blood into the bloodstream via direct contact with HIV infected blood or tissues. This can occur during transfusion of HIV infected blood or blood products, sexual contact, or sharing of needles or syringes. Healthcare workers (HCWs) can become infected occupationally as a result of a sharps/splash injury.

Infants born to women infected with HIV can become infected *in utero* and during birth due to contact with HIV infected blood and amniotic fluid. HIV infection can also be passed from mother to baby after birth during breast-feeding. Between 15 and 30% of babies born to HIV infected mothers become infected with HIV without intervention; this can be reduced to 1–2% with appropriate management, including antenatal care and screening, antiretroviral treatment, management of labour and avoidance of breast-feeding.

There is no risk of transmission of HIV infection during normal social and domestic contact with an HIV infected person.

INFECTIOUS PERIOD　A person infected with HIV is infectious shortly after infection and remains infectious for the rest of their lives. Everyone is susceptible to HIV infection except a very small minority of individuals with natural genetic resistance.

INFECTION CONTROL PRECAUTIONS

1 Isolation	Not required unless the patient is bleeding or is at risk of bleeding
2 Hand washing	Required
3 Gloves	Required for contact with blood and body fluids
4 Apron	Required for contact with blood and body fluids
5 Mask	A surgical mask should be worn if there is a risk of splashing of blood/body fluids
6 Eye protection	Required if there is a risk of splashing of blood/body fluids
7 Disinfection	Blood/body fluid spillage should be disinfected with chlorine-based products at 10 000 parts per million available chlorine strength

STAFF　The risk of becoming infected with HIV from an HIV infected patient following a sharps injury is three per 1000 injuries. Following splash injury the risk is less than one per 1000 injuries.

Needles used in an artery or vein, hollow needles and needles visibly stained with blood provide the greatest risk of transmission of infection, as do deep needlestick injuries and needlestick injuries where the source patient is terminally ill with a high viral load.

In terms of HIV transmission, the following body fluids are high risk: blood, semen, vaginal secretions, cerebrospinal fluid, synovial fluid, human breast milk, amniotic fluid, blood from body cavities and blood stained saliva, tissues and organs. Faeces, vomit, urine and saliva are low risk unless visibly blood stained.

Great care should be taken when there is a risk of contact with blood or body fluids, as it is then that the risk of transmission of infection is greatest. Safe sharps practice and disposal of sharps at the point of use reduces the likelihood of needlestick injury. Eye and, if necessary, full face protection must be worn if there is a risk of blood/body fluid splashes during a procedure.

In the event of a sharps injury, where inoculation with HIV infected blood/body fluids occurs, the affected area should be gently 'milked' to encourage a few drops of blood to flow, washed under running water and a dressing applied. Do not squeeze, suck or scrub the area. This is because chemical or physical trauma to the injury will cause inflammation and lead to increased numbers of white blood cells at the site, so increasing the likelihood of HIV infection. Attend Occupational Health or Accident and Emergency without delay. A risk assessment will be carried out to decide if post-exposure prophylaxis (PEP) is required. See the next subsection for further information on PEP.

In the event of a splash injury (where HIV infected blood/body fluids enters the eyes, mouth or nose) immediately rinse the affected area with copious amounts of water. Do not swallow this water. Attend Occupational Health or Accident and Emergency without delay. A risk assessment will be carried out to decide if PEP is required.

POST-EXPOSURE PROPHYLAXIS   PEP should ideally be started within one hour of the sharps/splash injury occurring and continued for four weeks. PEP can be commenced up to two weeks after the injury.

Whilst awaiting follow-up after PEP, providing seroconversion has not occurred, HCWs exposed to HIV infection can continue to work as normal. They should practice safe sex and should not donate blood during the follow-up period.

PEP can be given safely in pregnancy under expert advice.

VISITORS   Should adopt the same precautions as staff.

PATIENT TRANSFER   No special precautions are required. Inform the receiving ward/ department of the patient's HIV infection prior to transfer.

MORE INFORMATION   HIV infection is permanent and leads to severe immunosuppression, making the sufferer vulnerable to opportunistic infections, neoplasms and acquired immune deficiency syndrome (AIDS).

HIV transmission is particularly efficient in homosexual men. Receptive anal intercourse and multiple sexual partners are risk factors. Multiple sexual partners and sexually transmitted infections that cause genital ulcers are associated with the highest rates of infection in countries where heterosexual spread is common.

Highly active antiretroviral treatment (HAART) is very effective in treating HIV and most patients can expect to live an almost normal life-span in good health; it is not curative.

Impetigo

A superficial skin infection, usually confined to the face, seen most commonly in children. It is caused by *Staphylococcus aureus* or Group A streptococcus, often mixed.

SPREAD BY   Direct person-to-person contact. Indirect contact, e.g. through shared towels, clothes or toys. Outbreaks are common in schools and nurseries.

INFECTIOUS PERIOD   A patient should be considered infectious until 48 hours of appropriate antibiotic therapy have been completed. Precautions can then be stepped down.

INFECTION CONTROL PRECAUTIONS

1	Isolation	Required
2	Hand washing	Required
3	Gloves	Required
4	Apron	Required
5	Mask	Not required
6	Eye protection	Not required

STAFF   No further precautions.

VISITORS   Visitors must be reminded to perform hand hygiene after visiting. Newborn babies should not visit.

PATIENT TRANSFER   This should be kept to a minimum for the first 48 hours of treatment and the receiving ward/department must be informed of the diagnosis.

MORE INFORMATION   Clinical features are vesicles (fluid-filled blisters) on the skin around the mouth, that later become purulent with golden crusts.

Risk factors for impetigo include young age, nasal carriage of *S. aureus* and broken skin due either to minor trauma or to underlying skin problems such as eczema.

Impetigo is easily treated with antibiotics, either topical (cream or ointment) or systemic antibiotics such as flucloxacillin.

Influenza

Influenza or 'flu' is a respiratory infection caused by the influenza virus. Influenza infection may be classified as:

* Seasonal flu – the commonest kind of infection. Influenza is usually a winter infection that peaks between December and March in the northern hemisphere.
* Pandemic flu – worldwide outbreak of influenza that occurs when a new strain of influenza virus emerges
* Animal-related flu – animals, such as birds and pigs, get influenza too and can sometimes transmit this to people. This is uncommon but potentially serious.

The guidance below is applicable to all types of influenza. Always inform the Infection Prevention and Control Team of suspected influenza cases.

SPREAD BY   direct contact (e.g. touching the hands of a patient who has coughed into their hands).
* indirect contact (e.g. touching a door knob contaminated with virus).
* droplet spread (droplets of respiratory secretions entering the mouth/nose of those coming within one metre of the coughing/sneezing patient).
* airborne spread during aerosolising procedures.

Influenza virus has been shown to persist on environmental surfaces for up to 24 hours. Good hand hygiene and environmental cleaning are essential to limit transmission. Respiratory hygiene (see Chapter 2) is also important for patients, visitors and staff.

INFECTIOUS PERIOD   The incubation period for influenza is 1–4 days. Patients become infectious a day before their symptoms start and the infectious period lasts for as long as symptoms persist up to a maximum of 7 days. Isolation precautions can usually be discontinued after symptoms have resolved. Testing for viral clearance is not usually required. Patients who are immunocompromised or seriously ill may remain infectious for longer periods. Discuss with your Infection Prevention and Control Team if required.

INFECTION CONTROL PRECAUTIONS

1	Isolation	Required. Single room preferable. Cohorting is acceptable during pandemics
2	Hand washing	Required
3	Gloves	Required
4	Apron	Required
5	Mask	Required – see below for details
6	Eye protection	Not required unless aerosol-generating procedure

Isolation should be in a side room with the door closed and with personal protective equipment (PPE) available outside the door. Any non-essential items (furniture or equipment) should be removed before the patient arrives, to reduce clutter, which could impede cleaning. All staff and visitors should perform hand hygiene and wear PPE to enter the room, then remove PPE and perform hand hygiene when they leave the room.

Cohorting (managing patients with the same diagnosis together in a bay, rather than in individual side rooms) is acceptable during influenza pandemics. Ideally the diagnosis should be laboratory-confirmed, but in a pandemic the diagnosis may be based on clinical/epidemiological information.

Masks should be worn when working within 1 metre of a symptomatic patient – in practice we recommend wearing a mask at all times within cohorted areas or side rooms. Fluid-repellent surgical masks are adequate for general use. The mask should be replaced once it becomes moist or damaged. FFP3 respirator-style masks are only required for aerosol-generating procedures.

Gowns may be worn in place of aprons if extensive soiling of clothing or exposure to blood and body fluids is anticipated; if the gown is not fluid-repellent, wear a plastic apron underneath.

Cleaning should be escalated so that patient areas are cleaned at least daily, preferably more frequently, with a focus on frequently touched surfaces such as door knobs. The patient area should be cleaned thoroughly after discharge. Cleaners in an influenza room or bay should wear apron, gloves and surgical mask, then remove these and perform hand hygiene when they leave the area.

Equipment should ideally be either disposable or allocated to an influenza patient or cohort. If it must be shared, it should be cleaned with a detergent wipe before use on another patient.

Contact bays where a case of influenza has developed and other patients have been exposed are managed as follows: the index case is isolated in a side room and their bed space cleaned; the bay is closed to admissions for 7 days and reopened only if all contacts are asymptomatic; cleaning is escalated. Discuss with your Infection Prevention and Control Team.

Aerosol-generating procedures such as bronchoscopy (see Glossary) carry increased risk of infection via the aerosol route and so gown, gloves, eye protection and FFP3 mask should be worn by all staff present in the room during such a procedure.

STAFF   Staff should all be vaccinated against influenza annually, in order to protect themselves from influenza and also to prevent them transmitting influenza within the healthcare setting. Pregnant staff should ideally not care directly for patients with influenza. Staff who have been in contact with influenza should discuss with Occupational Health but are not usually restricted from working. Staff who have symptoms of influenza infection should not attend work and should inform Occupational Health. They can return to work once they have been asymptomatic for 48 hours.

Staff who are likely to care for influenza patients undergoing aerosol-generating procedures (e.g. staff on intensive care units or respiratory wards) should receive training in mask fit testing, which is important to ensure correct fitting of FFP3 masks. This can be done in advance of the influenza season.

VISITORS   Visitors should be kept to a minimum, ideally one designated visitor for the duration of their illness. Pregnant women, immunocompromised people and children should be discouraged from visiting. Visitors should perform hand hygiene and wear PPE to enter the room, then remove PPE and perform hand hygiene when they leave the room. Visitors to influenza patients should not visit other patients, mix with other patients' relatives or spend time in communal waiting areas. They should not visit if they develop symptoms of respiratory tract infection.

PATIENT TRANSFER   This should be kept to a minimum. The receiving ward/department should be informed of their diagnosis. The patient should wear a surgical face mask during transfer; if this is not possible they should follow respiratory hygiene measures. The patient should not wait in a communal waiting area. If going for an investigation or procedure, they should be placed last on the list to allow for cleaning/decontamination afterwards.

MORE INFORMATION   Common symptoms of influenza infection include fever, sore throat, runny nose, cough, headache, extreme tiredness and myalgia (muscle aches). Complications include secondary bacterial infections such as bronchitis and pneumonia. Patients with chronic underlying disease (lung, cardiac, renal, liver, neurological), who are immunosuppressed, or aged under 5 years or over 65 years of age, are at greater risk of these complications.

Investigation of influenza is performed on viral swabs of the nose or throat, or nasopharyngeal aspirate. PCR is now the standard method and results are usually available within 24–48 hours.

Prophylaxis and treatment with antiviral drugs such as oseltamivir is available but is not appropriate in every case. Discuss with your microbiologist.

Klebsiella

Klebsiella are bacteria that are normal flora of the intestine but can cause pneumonia, urinary tract infection, wound infection, IV line infection and bloodstream infection (bacteremia), and can also cause meningitis in neonates.

Outbreaks of infections can occur in hospitals, particularly in specialist units such as oncology or liver units.

Klebsiella are increasingly antibiotic resistant and some strains now produce ESBL (refer to the ESBL section if dealing with an ESBL-producing strain).

SPREAD BY   Direct spread on hands of staff.

INFECTIOUS PERIOD   This is likely to be indefinite, as *Klebsiella* is carried in the intestine, but carriage status is not usually assessed.

INFECTION CONTROL PRECAUTIONS

1	**Isolation**	Not required
2	**Hand washing**	Required
3	**Gloves**	Not required
4	**Apron**	Not required
5	**Mask**	Not required
6	**Eye protection**	Not required

STAFF   Good hand hygiene should control spread. No other restrictions.

VISITORS   No restrictions.

PATIENT TRANSFER   No restrictions.

MORE INFORMATION   There are several species of *Klebsiella* but there is no difference between the species in terms of treatment or infection control precautions.

Klebsiella are a genus of bacteria belonging to the coliform group.

Legionnaires disease

An infection caused by the waterborne bacterium *Legionella pneumophila*. May present as a febrile illness or an atypical pneumonia. Legionnaires disease is notifiable.

SPREAD BY Infection is acquired by exposure to aerosols of water containing *Legionella*. Outbreaks are often associated with water towers associated with cooling systems of large buildings or with spa pools. It is possible, though uncommon, to catch the infection in the domestic setting. Person-to-person transmission of *Legionella* does not occur.

INFECTIOUS PERIOD The incubation period is 2–19 days (usually 6 or 7 days). There is not a true infectious period because the infection is not spread from person to person.

INFECTION CONTROL PRECAUTIONS

1	Isolation	Not required
2	Hand washing	Required
3	Gloves	Not required
4	Apron	Not required
5	Mask	Not required
6	Eye protection	Not required

STAFF No further restrictions.

VISITORS No further restrictions.

PATIENT TRANSFER No restrictions.

MORE INFORMATION Any case of *Legionella* requires investigation to identify the source of infection. Symptoms include fever, myalgia, flu-like symptoms, dry cough, confusion and diarrhoea.

Diagnosis is by an antigen detection test on a urine sample, which is available in most laboratories as a same day test.

Treatment is with antibiotics, usually erythromycin or clarithromycin, with a second agent such as rifampicin for severe cases. Treatment is for 14 days.

Prevention and control of *Legionella* is a very topical issue and the focus is on ensuring water supplies are free from the bacteria. Most large buildings such as hospitals have complex plumbing and require expert advice on this. The mainstay is temperature control (cold water supply should be <20°C and hot water supply should be >60°C, as the bacteria prefer warm water and cannot grow at these extremes of temperature). In addition, low-use outlets should be identified and flushed regularly (usually for 5 minutes once a week) to prevent bacteria growing in stagnant water.

Legionella can be acquired at any stage of life but is more commonly seen in over-50s, males, smokers and the immunocompromised.

Leptospirosis (Weil's disease)

A multisystem disease caused by infection with the spirochaete bacterium *Leptospira interrogans*. Leptospirosis is no longer a notifiable disease, but the laboratory should notify the local Health Protection Unit if the diagnosis is laboratory-confirmed.

SPREAD BY   Infection is acquired by contact of broken skin or mucous membranes with urine of infected people or animals (most commonly rats or dogs, though any mammals may be affected). This includes contact with urine-contaminated water, which may occur occupationally (agriculture, sewage and abattoir workers) or recreationally (fishing, canoeing, other watersports). Person-to-person spread is extremely rare.

Leptospirosis is found all over the world, including the UK, but is commonest in tropical and subtropical regions.

INFECTIOUS PERIOD   The incubation period is 2–30 days (usually 7–21 days). Patients may remain infectious for up to a month after the onset of symptoms.

INFECTION CONTROL PRECAUTIONS

1	**Isolation**	Preferred
2	**Hand washing**	Required
3	**Gloves**	Required for contact with blood/body fluids
4	**Apron**	Required for contact with blood/body fluids
5	**Mask**	Required only for procedures where splashing of blood/body fluids may occur
6	**Eye protection**	Required only for procedures where splashing of blood/body fluids may occur

STAFF   No further restrictions.

VISITORS   No further restrictions.

PATIENT TRANSFER   No restrictions, though receiving ward/department must be informed of the diagnosis.

MORE INFORMATION   Symptoms
Infection may be asymptomatic, may cause a flu-like illness with severe headache and myalgia, or may cause a severe multisystem illness with jaundice, renal failure, red eyes, rash, meningism and widespread haemorrhages.

Prevention
Risk to water users can be minimised by these actions:

- Cover cuts with a waterproof plaster.
- Wear appropriate protective clothing.
- Shower promptly after water exposure, especially if you fall in.
- Avoid capsize drill or rolling in stagnant or slow moving water.
- Wear thick gloves when handling rats.
- Wash hands after animal handling and before eating.

Vaccination
This is not available in the UK. Antibiotic prophylaxis after exposure is not usually required.

Diagnosis
This is by blood cultures in the first 5 days of the illness, or serology (leptospiral IgM antibody detection) after 5 or more days.

Treatment
This is with doxycycline or benzylpenicillin.

Lice – head, body and pubic

Lice are parasitic insects (ectoparasites). There are many species of lice but only these three are clinically important. They present with itching. Lice or their eggs (nits) may be visible.

SPREAD BY   Close direct contact with an infested person. Sexual contact (pubic lice). Less commonly, transmission can occur via shared brushes, combs, clothing, bedding or towels.

INFECTIOUS PERIOD   Indefinite if untreated/have live lice on the head or body. The patient is much less infectious once they have been treated and clothing/linen changed and laundered. Patients with pubic lice are advised to avoid sexual contact until they have been treated and revaluated to rule out persistent infection.

INFECTION CONTROL PRECAUTIONS

1	**Isolation**	Not generally required, but preferred for head lice patients on paediatric wards
2	**Hand washing**	Required
3	**Gloves**	Not generally required, but wear gloves and apron to handle infested clothing and to apply chemical treatments
4	**Apron**	Not generally required (see above)
5	**Mask**	Not required
6	**Eye protection**	Not required

STAFF   Head-to-head contact with patients with head lice should be avoided as this can transmit the infestation. There is no risk of transmission of body or pubic lice to staff under standard working conditions.

VISITORS   Visitors should be kept to a minimum until the patient has been treated and should be discouraged from sitting on the bed or sharing any linen, towels, etc. Household/ close contacts of head lice patients are checked for lice and offered treatment if they have lice.

PATIENT TRANSFER   This should be kept to a minimum until the patient has been treated. The receiving ward/department should be informed of the diagnosis.

LINEN   Clothing, bedding and towels can spread infestation with body or pubic lice (or rarely with head lice). These items should not be shared. They should be treated as infected linen (red bag) or else machine washed at 60°C and dried at the high heat setting. Items that cannot be machine washed should be dry cleaned or else should be discarded.

COMBS AND BRUSHES   Those from a patient with head lice should be soaked in hot water (at least 60°C) for 5–10 minutes.

MORE INFORMATION
Head louse (*Pediculus humanus capitis*)
These lice are found on hair, most commonly behind the ears and at the back of the neck, rarely on eyelashes or eyebrows. The eggs (nits), baby lice (nymphs) or adult lice may be seen on the hair. Head lice are transmitted to another host when two heads are in close contact for 30 seconds or more, allowing the lice to crawl on to the next head. Preschool/primary school children and their families are most likely to have head lice, and

outbreaks are common in schools. Treatment is with wet combing or with chemical treatments such as malathion (apply, allow contact time of 8–12 hours and repeat treatment after 7 days in case any eggs survived the first application).

Body louse (Pediculus humanus corporis)

These lice usually infest people with poor personal hygiene. They live in the clothing but return to the skin to feed. The mainstay of treatment is regular bathing and clothing changes (at least once a week). Chemical treatments such as permethrin or malathion can be used: apply all over the body, wash off after 12 hours and repeat after 7 days.

Pubic louse (Phthirus pubis)

These live on coarse body hair, usually pubic but also facial (including eye lashes), axilla and chest hair. Permethrin or malathion are used to treat; wash and dry the affected area, then apply the medication, wash off after 12 hours and repeat the treatment after 7 days. Pubic lice are a sexually transmitted infection and so patients should be referred for a sexual health screen and partner notification.

Listeria

Caused by infection with the bacterium *Listeria monocytogenes*. Infection is usually asymptomatic or causes mild gastroenteritis or flu-like symptoms. In high-risk groups it can cause miscarriage, meningitis, bacteraemia and deep-seated infections such as abscesses.

Listeria infection is a notifiable disease.

SPREAD BY   Consumption of contaminated food, such as soft cheeses, patés, cold cuts of meat or inadequately heated cook-chill food. Vertical transmission from mother to baby may occur *in utero*, during birth or direct person-to-person spread soon after delivery.

INFECTIOUS PERIOD   The incubation period ranges from 3 to 70 days (average 30 days). Patients may carry *Listeria* in the gut for long periods, but for practical purposes they are unlikely to be infectious – person-to-person spread does not occur except from mother to baby.

INFECTION CONTROL PRECAUTIONS

1	**Isolation**	Preferred; essential if diarrhoea present
2	**Hand washing**	Required
3	**Gloves**	Required if diarrhoea present
4	**Apron**	Required if diarrhoea present
5	**Mask**	Not required
6	**Eye protection**	Not required

STAFF   No further precautions.

VISITORS   No further precautions.

PATIENT TRANSFER   No restrictions.

MORE INFORMATION   *Listeria* is widespread in the environment and is found in soil, raw food, sewage and in the gut of many animals, including farm animals. About 5% of the population have faecal carriage of *Listeria*, which is probably transient carriage following ingestion.

Listeria food poisoning is usually associated with ready-to-eat refrigerated and processed foods, because *Listeria* can survive and multiply at 4 °C.

Groups most at risk of serious *Listeria* infection include pregnant women, neonates, the elderly and the immunocompromised (including cancer, AIDS, alcoholism).

Control measures for *Listeria* centre around good food storage and handling, and avoidance of high-risk foods for susceptible groups.

Malaria

Malaria is a serious tropical disease that is spread by mosquito bites. Malaria is a notifiable disease.

SPREAD BY   Malaria is spread by the bite of the female *Anopheles* mosquito in countries where malaria is endemic. Malaria is found in Africa, Asia, South and Central America and the Middle East. Up to date maps of malaria distribution can be found on the WHO or NaTHNaC websites.

Malaria cannot be transmitted person to person. The only occasions where this has happened have been in healthcare facilities where basic infection control measures have been breached (e.g. using the same syringe of saline to flush IV lines on multiple patients).

INFECTIOUS PERIOD   Not applicable as person-to-person spread does not occur. The incubation period is at least 6 days but may be up to 6 months for falciparum infection or may be years for vivax and ovale infections.

INFECTION CONTROL PRECAUTIONS

1	Isolation	Not required
2	Hand washing	Required
3	Gloves	Not required
4	Apron	Not required
5	Mask	Not required
6	Eye protection	Not required

STAFF   No extra precautions required.

VISITORS   No extra precautions required.

PATIENT TRANSFER   This should not be restricted, but the receiving ward/department should be informed of the diagnosis.

MORE INFORMATION   The causative organism is the *Plasmodium* parasite, which invades red blood cells. There are several species of *Plasmodium*: *P. falciparum* causes the most severe infections and accounts for most hospitalised cases; *P. vivax, P. ovale* and *P. malariae* also affect humans, who can usually be treated as outpatients.

There are 1500–2000 travel-associated cases in the UK each year and 5–20 deaths.

Measles

Measles is a common and highly infectious childhood illness that may affect any age group. It is caused by the measles virus. Measles is a notifiable disease.

SPREAD BY

- Droplet spread – breathing in droplets expelled from an infected person when they cough/sneeze.
- Direct contact with nasal or throat secretions of infected persons.
- Indirect contact, e.g. by contact with objects freshly contaminated with nasal or throat secretions.

INFECTIOUS PERIOD   It has an incubation period of 7–18 days (average 10–12 days). Individuals are considered to be infectious from 1 day before prodromal symptoms (usually about 4 days before rash appears) to 4 days after the onset of the rash.

INFECTION CONTROL PRECAUTIONS

1	Isolation	Required
2	Hand washing	Required
3	Gloves	Required
4	Apron	Required
5	Mask	Required
6	Eye protection	Required only for procedures where splashing of blood/body fluids may occur

A patient with suspected measles, or any unidentified rash illness, should be kept out of the main waiting room or communal areas. Ideally they should be asked to attend at the end of surgery and/or wait in a side room.

STAFF   Staff looking after measles cases must have immunity to measles, either from two documented doses of MMR vaccine or from a history of measles infection that has been confirmed by positive serology. A list of staff, including ambulance staff, should be compiled and anyone who is not immune should be referred to Occupational Health for assessment. Pregnant staff members should be referred urgently if not immune.

VISITORS   Visitors should be kept to a minimum and should ideally be restricted during the infectious period to those with a history of measles infection or immunisation.

PATIENT TRANSFER   Patient transfer should be kept to a minimum and the receiving department/ward must be informed of the patient's condition. Patients must not wait in communal areas.

MORE INFORMATION   Measles is highly infectious. In general, 15 minutes in the same room as an infectious measles case, or face-to-face contact of any length, is enough to transmit infection. In immunosuppressed patients, even a very short exposure (minutes) may be sufficient to cause infection.

Any patient with suspected measles should be kept away from vulnerable contacts (immunosuppressed, pregnant, infants). Vulnerable contacts who have been exposed should be discussed as soon as possible with Microbiology or the Health Protection Unit in order to assess whether post-exposure prophylaxis with MMR or immunoglobulin is required.

Diagnosis is largely clinical but can be confirmed by oral fluid testing (arranged by the notification process) or serology.

Previously unimmunised cases should be fully immunised with MMR once recovered, ideally about 4 weeks after onset, in order to protect against the other infections.

Meningitis

Infection of the meninges (the membranes that surround the brain and spinal cord). Symptoms include fever, headache, photophobia and neck stiffness. Acute meningitis is a notifiable disease.

There are a variety of causes:

Bacterial meningitis
 Neisseria meningitidis (meningococcus)
 Streptococcus pneumoniae (pneumococcus)
 Haemophilus influenzae type B (Hib)
 Group B streptococcus in neonates
 Listeria in children and the elderly
 Rarely, other organisms
Viral meningitis – enterovirus, herpes simplex virus, rarely others
Tuberculous meningitis – TB
Fungal meningitis

SPREAD BY   Many different organisms can cause meningitis and their behaviour and routes of spread are not all identical. Your Infection Prevention Control Team will advise you on case management based upon laboratory results.

Neisseria meningitidis, the commonest bacterial cause of meningitis in the UK, is present in the nasopharynx and respiratory secretions of colonised or infected people. The bacteria are transmitted directly during close face-to-face contact or aerosol-generating procedures, and therefore close household or 'kissing contacts' are most at risk of transmission. They may also spread indirectly by respiratory secretions contaminating surfaces.

Streptococcus pneumoniae and *Haemophilus influenzae* are also transmitted via respiratory secretions.

Less often, a head or middle ear injury may allow direct spread of bacteria from the patient's own ear/nose/throat into the meninges.

Viral meningitis may be spread by faecal–oral transmission (enterovirus) or by close direct contact (herpes simplex). Viral meningitis is not considered easily transmissible, although viral meningitis patients are isolated if possible.

TB meningitis often follows chronic TB infection.

Fungal meningitis is not spread from person to person. It generally follows a fungal bloodstream infection in an immunocompromised person.

INFECTIOUS PERIOD   Bacterial meningitis is considered infectious until 24 hours after antibiotics are given.

INFECTION CONTROL PRECAUTIONS

1	Isolation	Required for first 24 hours
2	Hand washing	Required
3	Gloves	Required for first 24 hours
4	Apron	Required for first 24 hours
5	Mask	Only required for aerosol generating procedures (subject to local agreement)
6	Eye protection	Not required

STAFF   Most staff caring for a meningitis patient will not require any prophylaxis, provided the infection control measures above have been followed. The exception would be healthcare workers who have been exposed to infected respiratory droplets/secretions within a 1 metre radius of a patient with probable or confirmed meningococcal infection before the patient has completed 24 hours of antibiotics. This scenario is most likely to occur in staff who have performed airway management during resuscitation without wearing a mask. If this has occurred, discuss with your Occupational Health Department.

VISITORS   Visitors should be limited to essential visitors only for the first 24 hours, partly to limit exposure but also to allow the patient to rest. Visitors should be asked to comply with full infection control precautions for the first 24 hours of treatment.

PATIENT TRANSFER   This should be limited to essential transfers only for the first 24 hours. The receiving ward/department must be informed of their condition.

MORE INFORMATION   The Health Protection Agency will advise on contact tracing and prophylaxis as required. Close (household or kissing) contacts of bacterial meningitis may be offered antibiotic prophylaxis, usually a single dose of ciprofloxacin.

Effective vaccines exist against many of the bacterial causes of meningitis: *N. meningitidis* (Groups C and ACWY), *H. influenzae, S. pneumoniae* and TB. No vaccine is yet available for *N. meningitidis* Group B. Meningitis C, pneumococcal and Hib vaccination are part of the routine childhood immunisation programme in the UK.

Methicillin-resistant *Staphylococcus aureus* (MRSA)

MRSA is a type of *Staphylococcus aureus* that is resistant to methicillin (a penicillin) and to other commonly used antibiotics. Like *S. aureus*, it may colonise people without causing illness or may cause clinical infection. MRSA bloodstream infection (bacteraemia) was once considered a hospital-acquired infection; however it is increasingly common in the community.

SPREAD BY   Many MRSA infections are autoinfections, i.e. the patient's own colonising flora causing an infection. This is particularly likely if there is a break in the skin, such as minor trauma or a leg ulcer. MRSA may also be transmitted from person to person via the hands of healthcare workers, via dirty or dusty equipment and via airborne spread, e.g. from clouds of MRSA dispersed during bedmaking.

INFECTIOUS PERIOD   Indefinite. Patients with MRSA may carry it in a variety of sites such as nose, axilla, groin, elsewhere on the skin and even in the gut. This makes it difficult to eradicate reliably. Even if MRSA decolonisation has been performed and negative screens achieved, the MRSA may reappear at a later date. Speak to your Infection Prevention and Control Team before stepping down infection control precautions.

INFECTION CONTROL PRECAUTIONS   Ideally these precautions should be put in place for all patients. In practice, if insufficient side rooms are available then a risk assessment may be used to prioritise side room use, giving precedence to patients/clinical areas where there is a high risk of acquiring MRSA infection or where MRSA infection would have serious consequences. For example, orthopaedic and surgical patients with MRSA should always be isolated, whereas medical patients are sometimes managed in the open ward.

1	Isolation	Required
2	Hand washing	Required
3	Gloves	Required
4	Apron	Required
5	Mask	Not required
6	Eye protection	Not required

STAFF   Staff compliance with hand hygiene is the single most important action to prevent the spread of MRSA. Staffing levels must be adequate to allow time for hand hygiene. Screening of staff is not common practice but may be considered if there is an outbreak of MRSA infections in a clinical area. Transient carriage of MRSA after caring for an MRSA-positive patient is common but is generally lost within a day and carries little risk of onward transmission, so if screening is considered it should be done at the start rather than the end of a shift.

VISITORS   Visitors should perform hand hygiene after visiting the patient.

PATIENT TRANSFER   Patient transfer is permitted, but the receiving ward/department must be informed in advance that they are MRSA-positive. If going for a procedure they should be last on the list to allow for cleaning afterwards.

EQUIPMENT AND THE ENVIRONMENT   These must be kept clean, as MRSA survives in dust. The environment should be kept uncluttered and cleaned regularly during the patient's stay. After the patient leaves, a thorough clean should be performed, which includes: thorough washing of all horizontal surfaces and equipment with warm soapy water and disposal of all disposable items. If curtains have become contaminated (i.e. through hands of healthcare workers) these should be removed and laundered.

Equipment should either be for single patient use or should be cleaned with detergent before use on another patient.

SCREENING FOR MRSA   This is performed before many elective procedures and for most emergency admissions. Swabs should be taken from the nose (one swab for both nostrils), skin lesions/wounds/tracheostomy, catheter urine if a catheter is present, groin/perineum and sputum from patients with a productive cough. Many hospitals also swab the throat. Swabs should be moistened in sterile saline before using on the patient, as a moistened swab picks up more bacteria than a dry swab, which increases the sensitivity of the test. A positive screen should be dealt with according to local protocol (see below).

DECOLONISATION FOR MRSA   This concerns the use of topical agents such as nasal ointment, body wash and shampoo to reduce nasal/skin carriage of MRSA. It does not always completely eradicate MRSA but will reduce the bioburden, which in turn reduces the risk of transmission and of surgical wound infection.

Each individual patient must be assessed fully before specific treatments are prescribed. Inappropriate use must be avoided to reduce the likelihood of resistance occurring. Decolonisation is much less likely to succeed in a patient with wounds, skin lesions or indwelling medical devices (catheters, IV lines, etc.).

Decolonisation protocols last for 5 days. The timing of the protocol is important:

- Five days of decolonisation immediately for inpatients.
- Five days of decolonisation immediately for prospective orthopaedic surgery patients, followed by three negative screens taken at least 48 hours apart before they are considered for surgery.
- General surgical patients can usually have their 5 days of decolonisation given in the 5 days leading up to the procedure, with no need for rescreening.

A typical decolonisation programme includes:

Nasal decolonisation: mupirocin 2% in a paraffin base. Apply a small pea-sized amount to the inner surface of each nostril using a cotton bud or clean fingertip and massage backward until the patient can taste it in their throat. Three times daily for 5 days.

Skin decolonisation: using an antiseptic detergent such as 4% chlorhexidine, 7.5% povidone iodine or other products as agreed locally. The patient should bathe or shower daily for 5 days, moistening the skin first, then applying the detergent all over (including hair) before washing it all off.

Clean clothing, bedding and towels should ideally be used after each wash.

Throat carriage of MRSA is very difficult to eradicate and this should only be undertaken on the advice of a consultant microbiologist. The presence of dentures makes mouth and throat clearance difficult as MRSA adheres to synthetic material.

It is important that all colonised/infected areas are treated simultaneously and treatments are correctly applied.

Decolonisation protocols initiated in the acute hospital should always be completed following transfer of the patient into the community setting.

MORE INFORMATION   Like *S. aureus*, MRSA can cause a range of infections including:

- skin and soft tissue infections (SSTI) such as impetigo, cellulitis, paronychia, abscesses;
- conjunctivitis;
- wound and IV line infections;
- pneumonia;
- deep-seated infections such as osteomyelitis, septic arthritis, endocarditis;
- toxic shock syndrome;
- bacteraemia.

MRSA infections are no more aggressive than other *S. aureus* infections, but they are more difficult to manage because there are fewer antibiotic treatment options. Diagnosis is by microscopy and culture and treatment requires drainage of pus, removal of foreign bodies, where possible, and antibiotic treatment if clinically necessary.

Multiresistant bacteria

Bacteria may be intrinsically resistant to antibiotics or may acquire resistance, usually as a result of being exposed to antibiotics (antibiotic pressure). Antibiotic resistance has two practical implications:

1. Infections with a resistant organism are more difficult to treat and often require antibiotics that are more toxic and more expensive.
2. Infection control must be enhanced to prevent spread of resistant organisms to the environment, staff and other patients.

SPREAD BY   The route of spread varies between organisms, but a general principle for multiresistant organisms in healthcare settings is that they can be transferred on the hands of staff and thus on to patients or into the environment (where they may later be transferred on to patients).

Therefore the methods of control are isolation and hand hygiene (see below). The environment must be kept clean and uncluttered to minimise contamination.

INFECTIOUS PERIOD   This depends on the organism. Many multiresistant organisms are carried indefinitely, particularly those that are present in the intestine ('gut carriage'), such as ESBL and VRE. Infection control precautions should be continued indefinitely unless the Infection Prevention and Control Team advise otherwise.

Further details are available under the organism name in this A–Z.

INFECTION CONTROL PRECAUTIONS

1 Isolation	Required
2 Hand washing	Required
3 Gloves	Required
4 Apron	Required
5 Mask	Not required
6 Eye protection	Not required

STAFF/VISITORS   Further advice/precautions depend on the exact nature of the organism.

PATIENT TRANSFER   Patient transfer should only occur if clinically necessary and the receiving ward/department must be made aware of the diagnosis.

MORE INFORMATION   Antibiotic resistance was identified by the World Health Organisation in 2009 as one of the three greatest threats to human health. An estimated 25000 people die in the European Union each year from antibiotic-resistant bacterial infections. Increasing antibiotic resistance could mean that many routine procedures and operations will not be possible in the future, and that morbidity and mortality from untreatable infections will rise.

Examples of resistant organisms include:

- Methicillin-resistant *Staphylococcus aureus* (MRSA)
- Vancomycin-resistant *Enterococcus* (VRE), also known as glycopeptide-resistant *Enterococcus* (GRE)
- Extended spectrum beta lactamase (ESBL) inhibitors
- Carbapenemase producers (resistant to meropenem and imipenem)

- Multiresistant *Acinetobacter baumanii* (MRAB)
- Penicillin-resistant *Streptococcus pneumoniae*
- Antibiotic-resistant gonorrhoea

In addition, other organisms that have an unusually resistant antibiogram (antibiotic sensitivity test results), such as a gentamicin-resistant *E. coli*, may be treated as being multiresistant. Your microbiologist will advise as required.

Risk factors for carriage of multiresistant organisms include:

- Multiple or prolonged courses of antibiotics
- Multiple or prolonged hospital admissions
- History of healthcare in other countries*
- History of residence in other countries*

*Many other countries have unrestricted antibiotic use and therefore have high rates of antibiotic resistance. Examples are Asia, Greece and Southern Europe.

Good antibiotic stewardship will reduce antibiotic pressure and thus slow the spread of multiresistant bacteria.

Mumps

Mumps is an acute viral illness caused by infection with mumps virus. Mumps is a notifiable disease.

SPREAD BY

* Droplet transmission.
* Direct contact (with the saliva of an infected person, e.g. sharing food or drinks).
* Indirect contact (e.g. hands touching a contaminated surface and then touching the eyes, nose or mouth).

INFECTIOUS PERIOD   The incubation period is 14–21 days. Patients are infectious from several days before the parotid swelling until 5 days after symptoms appear.

People are considered susceptible (non-immune) if they have no clear history of mumps and have not had two doses of mumps vaccine.

Exposed non-immune people are considered potentially infectious from the 12th through to the 25th day after exposure.

INFECTION CONTROL PRECAUTIONS

1	Isolation	Required
2	Hand washing	Required
3	Gloves	Required
4	Apron	Required
5	Mask	Not required
6	Eye protection	Not required

STAFF   Staff should be immune to or vaccinated against mumps. Screening for mumps immunity is usually done by Occupational Health on recruitment. Staff who have been in contact with a case of mumps are usually allowed to continue work. If they do not have two documented doses of MMR they should seek advice from Occupational Health. If they are non-immune and develop fever or any symptoms of mumps they should stay away from work and discuss with Occupational Health. Staff who have symptoms of mumps infection should be excluded from work for 5 days from the onset of symptoms.

VISITORS   Visitors should be limited to one or two essential visitors and should wear PPE as above and perform hand hygiene. Non-immune people should not visit.

PATIENT TRANSFER   Patient transfer should be kept to a minimum. The receiving ward/ department should be informed of the diagnosis. The patient should wear a surgical mask/ comply with respiratory hygiene during transfer.

MORE INFORMATION   Symptoms of mumps include headache, fever, swelling of parotid glands (unilateral or bilateral), abdominal and testicular pain. Mumps may be asymptomatic in 30% of cases.

Complications of mumps include viral meningitis, deafness, orchitis, oophoritis and pancreatitis.

The diagnosis can be confirmed by oral fluid testing (arranged via the notification process) or serology.

Mumps can occur year-round but cases peak in the winter and spring in the United Kingdom.

Mumps is a vaccine-preventable disease. The mumps virus vaccine is incorporated in the MMR vaccine, which is a standard childhood immunisation.

Necrotising fasciitis

This is a severe, often fatal, soft tissue infection involving the dermis, subcutaneous fat and superficial fascia. Infection has an acute onset and may progress very rapidly. The cause is classically Group A streptococcus but can be a mixed infection with coliforms and anaerobes, particularly in post-surgical infections or infections of the male genitalia (known as Fournier's gangrene).

SPREAD BY   Autoinfection (infection by patient's own flora) is the commonest route of spread. Group A streptococcus may also be spread by direct person-to-person spread or indirect spread via fomites.

Necrotising fasciitis is not easily 'caught' but affected patients should be isolated until they have completed at least 24 hours of antibiotics and they have shown clinical improvement.

INFECTIOUS PERIOD   Generally up to 24 hours after antibiotic treatment is commenced, but depends on the causative bacterium.

INFECTION CONTROL PRECAUTIONS

1	Isolation	Required for minimum first 24 hours of treatment (longer if necessary, until patient is clinically improving)
2	Hand washing	Required
3	Gloves	Required for contact with blood/body fluids
4	Apron	Required for contact with blood/body fluids
5	Mask	Required only for procedures where splashing of blood/body fluids may occur
6	Eye protection	Required only for procedures where splashing of blood/body fluids may occur

STAFF   No further restrictions.

VISITORS   Limit visitor numbers for the first 24 hours and follow infection control precautions as above. Ask them for details of household contacts to assist the Health Protection team with their management.

PATIENT TRANSFER   Patient transfer should ideally be kept to a minimum for the first 24 hours of treatment, but this should not be allowed to delay treatment. Receiving wards/departments must be informed of the diagnosis.

MORE INFORMATION   The local Health Protection Unit should be informed of confirmed cases of invasive Group A streptococcal infection (iGAS).

Norovirus

Also previously known as 'winter vomiting disease', small round structured viruses (SRSV) and 'Norwalk' virus. Norovirus is the most common cause of infectious gastroenteritis in England and Wales and worldwide. It causes a short-lived but unpleasant illness: there is sudden onset of vomiting, diarrhoea and malaise, which usually resolves completely within two days.

SPREAD BY

1. Ingestion of foodstuffs that have become contaminated, e.g. food handled by a person infected with norovirus, raw or inadequately cooked shellfish grown in water contaminated with sewage.
2. Person-to-person spread through the faecal–oral route: norovirus is contained within vomit and faeces and when a person has diarrhoea, or vomits, droplets of diarrhoea and/or vomit containing the virus contaminate environmental surfaces, which, if not cleaned properly can lead to further spread.
3. Consumption of contaminated drinking water.
4. Swimming in contaminated water.

INFECTIOUS PERIOD   A person with norovirus is infectious from the onset of symptoms until 48 hours after their last episode of diarrhoea/vomiting.

INFECTION CONTROL PRECAUTIONS

1	Isolation	Required
2	Hand washing	Required – soap and water should be used, *not* alcohol handrub
3	Gloves	Required – must be changed after each patient with hands washed after removal
4	Apron	Required – must be changed after each patient with hands washed after removal
5	Mask	Not required unless there is a risk of splashing
6	Eye protection	Not required unless there is a risk of splashing

STAFF   Staff are at high risk of infection due to their contact with patients and a potentially contaminated environment. Hand hygiene is of utmost importance using soap and water. Staff who develop symptoms must go home and remain off work until 48 hours after their last episode of diarrhoea/vomiting.

VISITORS   Visitors should be restricted and children should be excluded from visiting. Visitors should adopt the same precautions as for staff.
It is important that visitors are educated in appropriate glove and apron use, i.e.:

- to remove them and clean their hands before leaving the isolated room/ bay;
- not to assist other patients whilst wearing aprons and gloves;
- not to leave the isolated room/bay that they are visiting whilst still wearing an apron and gloves;
- not to eat and drink in the isolated room/bay;
- not to prepare beverages or foodstuffs whilst wearing an apron and gloves.

PATIENT TRANSFER   Patients in a ward/bay that is closed to admissions due to norovirus must not be transferred to another part of the hospital unless there is an urgent clinical need. They must not be transferred to another institution, even if they are asymptomatic, as they could be incubating norovirus, which could lead to an outbreak in the receiving institution.

Any patient known or suspected to have norovirus:

- Should not be moved from their room/ward unless it is an emergency, as otherwise all other persons who come into contact with them are at risk of infection. If transfer is unavoidable the receiving ward/department must be informed that the patient is known or suspected to have norovirus, or that they are coming from a ward affected by norovirus.
- Requiring an urgent investigation should be seen last on the list if possible and after their treatment the environment must be cleaned and disinfected, before any other patients are treated there.
- Should not be transferred to another hospital/care home/residential institution whilst diarrhoea and/or vomiting symptoms are ongoing, as this could lead to an outbreak in the receiving institution.
- Can be discharged home to their own home providing they are medically fit and capable of looking after themself at home or have someone who can help them at home. It is important that they know to contact their GP (but not to attend the surgery) if their symptoms worsen or do not resolve within 2–3 days.

MORE INFORMATION   Norovirus has a very high attack rate and many people who come into contact with an infected person will become unwell themselves, including staff.

Norovirus is often diagnosed after the patient's symptoms have resolved; therefore it is essential that patients suspected to have norovirus are nursed in isolation in a single room or in a bay closed to admissions to prevent further spread.

If norovirus is suspected it is important to contact the Infection Prevention and Control Team before making any decisions about patient placement.

Norovirus can remain infectious in the environment on surfaces, carpets and curtains; therefore cleaning and disinfection are important to prevent further spread. To enable effective cleaning and disinfection it is essential that the environment is free of clutter. In a hospital ward it is important that rooms and bays (where isolation precautions are in place for norovirus) do not contain supplies of sheets, gowns, bedding, gloves, aprons, pads, etc., as these items can become contaminated through airborne contamination when a patient vomits or from contaminated hands.

Patient equipment must be cleaned after each use. Soapy water or detergent wipes are suitable for this and the environment should be disinfected with hypochlorite solution at 1000 parts per million (ppm) available chlorine.

Enhanced cleaning should be carried out when patients have norovirus. This involves cleaning and disinfecting the environment more frequently than once a day, with particular attention to items/areas that are touched frequently after using the toilet, i.e. toilets, commodes, taps, sinks, toilet flush handles, light switches, soap dispensers, door handles.

Patients must be given the opportunity to clean their hands after using the toilet/vomiting using soap and water.

Outbreaks of norovirus are reported to the Health Protection Agency by the Infection Prevention and Control Team.

Panton–Valentine leucocidin (PVL)

Panton–Valentine leucocidin (PVL) is a toxin produced by some strains (less than 2%) of MRSA and MSSA (methicillin-sensitive *Staphylococcus aureus*). The presence of PVL causes increased severity of infections, such as recurrent boils and abscesses, cellulitis and necrotising pneumonia. PVL is not a notifiable disease but the laboratory usually informs the local Health Protection Unit.

SPREAD BY   PVL is spread as part of MRSA/MSSA bacteria and therefore is transmitted in the same way, i.e. by:

Autoinfections, i.e. infections with the patient's own colonising flora
Direct person-to-person contact
Indirect contact, e.g. via dirty or dusty equipment
Airborne spread, e.g. from clouds of staphylococci dispersed during bedmaking

   PVL is not particularly associated with hospitals or healthcare. It is most frequently seen in young healthy people in the community. It may spread within groups or institutions where there is close contact, e.g. rugby clubs, boarding schools, gyms, etc. Risk factors for community transmission are described as the '5Cs':

* Contaminated items shared, e.g. towels, razors
* Close contact
* Crowding
* Cleanliness (poor hygiene) ·
* Cuts and other compromised skin integrity

INFECTIOUS PERIOD   Indefinite while patient remains colonised.

INFECTION CONTROL PRECAUTIONS

1	Isolation	Required
2	Hand washing	Required
3	Gloves	Required
4	Apron	Required
5	Mask	Not required, except during intubation/respiratory care of necrotising pneumonia
6	Eye protection	Not required, except during intubation/respiratory care of necrotising pneumonia

STAFF   No further restrictions. Staff who carry PVL should attend Occupational Health for advice and decolonisation. Staff with acute PVL infection must remain off work until clinically better and until 2 days of a 5-day decolonisation regime has been completed.

VISITORS   Visitors must wash their hands before and after visiting.

PATIENT TRANSFER   Patient transfer is permitted but should be kept to a minimum and the receiving ward/department must be informed of the diagnosis. Procedures should be done last on the list to allow for cleaning afterwards.

MORE INFORMATION   Panton and Valentine were the two doctors who discovered PVL. 'Leucocidin' means that it kills white blood cells. This feature is the reason why PVL infections are more serious, because the body's immune defences cannot work effectively.

PVL infections are managed by incision and drainage of skin lesions. Antibiotics are used as adjunctive treatment. Choice of antibiotics depends on sensitivity results.

Household and close contacts of PVL cases should be screened for PVL carriage with a swab of skin lesions and anterior nares (nose). Ensure that PVL is requested and that risk factors (e.g. household contact) are stated.

PVL cases and carriers should have a 5-day decolonisation treatment similar to MRSA decolonisation. This may be coordinated by the GP or by the Health Protection Unit. Decolonisation is best deferred until the clinical infection has resolved.

Parainfluenza

Human parainfluenza viruses are a group of RNA viruses that can cause respiratory infections, particularly in young children. Their significance in healthcare settings is that they can cause outbreaks of infection among immunocompromised patients, e.g. on haematology or oncology wards.

SPREAD BY   direct contact (e.g. touching the hands of a patient who has coughed into their hands);

* indirect contact (e.g. touching a door knob contaminated with virus);
* droplet spread (e.g. inhaling droplets of respiratory secretions immediately after a patient sneezes).

Control measures include good hand hygiene, respiratory hygiene (see Glossary) and regular cleaning.

INFECTIOUS PERIOD   The incubation period is 1–7 days. Patients become infectious the day before symptoms start and are considered infectious until they are asymptomatic for 48 hours. The average duration of illness is 7–10 days. Immunocompromised patients may remain infectious for longer – discuss with your Infection Prevention and Control team.

INFECTION CONTROL PRECAUTIONS

1	Isolation	Preferred on paediatric wards; required on wards where immunosuppressed patients present
2	Hand washing	Required
3	Gloves	Required
4	Apron	Required
5	Mask	Not required
6	Eye protection	Not required

It is always good practice to isolate patients with respiratory infections. Parainfluenza infection is not always regarded as serious, as most cases do not require hospital admission. However, it is preferable to isolate inpatients with parainfluenza and this is essential on wards with immunosuppressed patients or in an outbreak.

STAFF   No further precautions. No vaccine available.

VISITORS   Visitors should be restricted to one or two essential visitors. Visitors do not need to wear gloves and aprons, providing they only have contact with the person they are visiting. Visitors should perform hand hygiene before and after seeing the patient.

PATIENT TRANSFER   Patient transfer should be kept to a minimum. The receiving ward/department should be informed of their diagnosis. They should perform respiratory hygiene.

MORE INFORMATION   Symptoms range from mild to severe and include fever, cough, coryza (cold symptoms), croup, laryngitis, bronchitis, bronchiolitis and pneumonia.
   Not all hospitals test samples for parainfluenza virus, but the infection control precautions required are those that should be put in place for any respiratory infection.

Paratyphoid

A systemic infection with gastrointestinal symptoms, caused by infection with *Salmonella paratyphi*. It is also known as *Salmonella enterica* serovar paratyphi A, B and C. Paratyphoid resembles typhoid but is a milder illness. Paratyphoid is a notifiable disease.

SPREAD BY   The infection is present in the stools and sometimes in the blood and urine of an infected person. *S. paratyphi* B infections have rarely been associated with contact with cattle.

The commonest mode of spread is faecal–oral, usually through contaminated water (mainly in the developing world) or by contamination of food. Direct person-to-person faecal–oral transmission can occur in poor hygiene conditions or in men who have sex with men. Household transmission of infection may occur, probably through lapses in food hygiene. Most cases in the UK are acquired abroad.

INFECTIOUS PERIOD   The incubation period is 1–10 days. Most people excrete *S. paratyphi* and remain potentially infectious for 5–6 weeks. A small minority of cases become chronic carriers who continue to shed bacteria in the stool indefinitely.

INFECTION CONTROL PRECAUTIONS

1	Isolation	Required
2	Hand washing	Required
3	Gloves	Required
4	Apron	Required
5	Mask	Not required
6	Eye protection	Not required

STAFF   Staff should wear a mask if there is significant risk of splash to the face.

VISITORS   Visitors should be reminded not to eat or drink in the patient's room. They should wear PPE as above and should wash their hands when leaving the isolation room.

PATIENT TRANSFER   Patient transfer should only occur if necessary and the receiving ward/department must be informed of the diagnosis.

MORE INFORMATION   Infection with paratyphoid or typhoid is known as enteric fever.

Clinical features of paratyphoid include fever, myalgia, abdominal pain, diarrhoea and headache. Some patients have a rash on the trunk known as 'rose spots'.

Diagnosis is usually by stool sample, but blood or urine culture may also be positive. Serology is rarely useful.

Treatment is with antibiotics and depends upon sensitivity testing results: ciprofloxacin is the drug of choice if sensitive.

There is no vaccine against paratyphoid.

Parvovirus

Infection with parvovirus causes a common childhood disease sometimes called slapped cheek disease, Fifth disease or erythema infectiosum. Parvovirus can also affect adults.

SPREAD BY   Contact with infected respiratory secretions, transfusion of infected blood/ blood products or vertical (mother to child).

INFECTIOUS PERIOD   The incubation period is 13–18 days. Once the rash or joint pains appear, the patient is no longer infectious.

INFECTION CONTROL PRECAUTIONS

1	Isolation	Not required
2	Hand washing	Required
3	Gloves	Not required
4	Apron	Not required
5	Mask	Not required
6	Eye protection	Not required

Patients rarely present while still infectious and so isolation is not usually required. However, patients with haematological disorders such as sickle-cell disease or immunocompromised patients may be infectious when first admitted and may remain infectious for longer; their isolation should be discussed with the Infection Prevention and Control Team.

STAFF   Pregnant staff should ideally not care for patients with parvovirus or any other rash illness. The likelihood of a pregnant staff member acquiring parvovirus at work is extremely low.

VISITORS   Pregnant women should not visit in the early stage of the illness.

PATIENT TRANSFER   Patient transfer should be kept to a minimum while still infectious, but there are no restrictions once the rash has appeared.

MORE INFORMATION   Parvovirus infects red blood cell precursors and this explains why it can cause haematological complications.
   Clinical features are a facial rash most intense on the cheeks, spreading to the trunk and limbs. There may be non-specific flu-like symptoms, mild generalised lymphadenopathy and arthralgia. About 20% of cases are asymptomatic.
   Complications include aplastic crises in patients with pre-existing red cell problems such as sickle-cell anaemia or thalassaemia, infection in pregnancy and chronic anaemia in immunodeficiency.
   Pregnant women who may have been exposed to parvovirus should seek medical advice. Parvovirus infection in the first 20 weeks of pregnancy may lead to fetal abnormalities or anaemia, or miscarriage.
   Diagnosis is by serology (detection of parvovirus IgM).
   One infection with parvovirus is thought to confer lifelong immunity.

Pests and vermin

Healthcare facilities can encounter problems with some or all of the following pests: rats, mice, pigeons, squirrels, cockroaches, ants (including Pharoah's ants), flies and maggots, bed bugs and fleas.

These infestations are unacceptable to patients and the public. They may cause destruction to the buildings or to equipment such as sterile supplies, may taint and spoil food, and may in theory transmit infection.

SPREAD BY   Pests and vermin all require food, water and shelter and are more likely to be found in areas where these are available.

INFECTIOUS PERIOD   This is dependent on the particular pest. An infestation will remain a problem until the pest has been eradicated. Pests and vermin that carry disease affecting humans are an infection risk as long as they are present in the environment.

INFECTION CONTROL PRECAUTIONS

1	**Isolation**	Not required*
2	**Hand washing**	Required
3	**Gloves**	Required
4	**Apron**	Required
5	**Mask**	Not required
6	**Eye protection**	Not required

*Inpatient areas affected by pests or vermin should not be used until the pest has been removed/eradicated. A patient with fleas should be isolated until their infested clothing has been removed (see subsection on 'fleas').

STAFF   No additional precautions are required.

VISITORS   No additional precautions are required.

PATIENT TRANSFER   No special precautions.

MORE INFORMATION

Preventing infestations

Eliminate food sources: keep food covered (preferably in pest-proof airtight containers), clear food debris immediately after meals, dispose of waste regularly and do not feed birds or animals.

Eliminate water sources: report any water leaks, ensure there are no pools of water, e.g. in cleaners' cupboards.

Eliminate shelter: the fabric of the building should be well maintained with no cracks and crevices or unsealed areas around pipework. Drains should be covered. Fly screens and bird netting may be required to prevent access. Do not allow clutter to accumulate.

Signs of infestation

Direct sighting of pests/vermin
Indirect sighting, i.e. discovery of droppings, nesting, gnawing

Action in the event of a problem

Notify your line manager or the Estates department immediately, giving details of the area and the nature of the problem. Most healthcare facilities have a pest control policy, which may be provided by an approved pest control contractor.

Pseudomonas

Pseudomonas are Gram-negative bacteria, which are common in the environment but which can cause clinical infection, particularly in people who have diabetes, burns, cystic fibrosis or who are immunocompromised. The most commonly encountered species is Pseudomonas aeruginosa.

SPREAD BY   Direct person-to-person contact. Indirect contact, e.g. on hands of staff or via contaminated equipment such as water reservoirs in respiratory equipment.

INFECTIOUS PERIOD   Indefinite. Pseudomonas can be carried in the gut and is therefore difficult to eradicate. Faecal carriage rates in the general population are 15–25%.

INFECTION CONTROL PRECAUTIONS   The level of precautions taken depends on the antibiotic resistance of the organism. In most cases, only standard precautions are required. If it is multiply antibiotic resistant then isolation may be required – your microbiologist should guide you.

1	Isolation	Not required
2	Hand washing	Required
3	Gloves	Not required
4	Apron	Not required
5	Mask	Not required
6	Eye protection	Not required

STAFF   No further precautions.

VISITORS   No further precautions.

PATIENT TRANSFER   No further restrictions.

MORE INFORMATION   Pseudomonas can cause a wide range of infections in susceptible patients, including hospital-acquired pneumonia, line infections, UTI, soft tissue infection and bacteremia.

Pseudomonas is intrinsically resistant to many antibiotics and can acquire further resistance under antibiotic pressure. Treatment options are frequently limited and choice of antibiotic should be guided by sensitivity testing.

In the healthcare setting, water supplies in augmented care units such as ITU should be tested regularly to ensure they are free from Pseudomonas and appropriate action must be taken if it is detected.

Rabies

This is a rare and serious viral infection caused by the rabies virus. Rabies is a notifiable disease.

SPREAD BY   Transmitted in the saliva of an infected animal, usually passed on via bites or scratches. Human-to-human transmission has never been shown to happen, except in rare cases involving organ transplantation from donors with undiagnosed rabies. There is a theoretical risk from exposure to an infected person's body fluids as the virus is present in saliva.

INFECTIOUS PERIOD   The incubation period is usually 2–8 weeks but can sometimes be several months or even years. The infectious period begins several days before the onset of symptoms and lasts for the duration of the illness.

INFECTION CONTROL PRECAUTIONS

1	Isolation	Required
2	Hand washing	Required
3	Gloves	Required
4	Apron	Required. Wear a gown if risk of splashing of blood/body fluids
5	Mask	Required only for procedures where splashing of blood/body fluids may occur
6	Eye protection	Required only for procedures where splashing of blood/body fluids may occur

STAFF   The number of staff in contact with the patient should be kept to a minimum. Rabies vaccination is not given routinely to staff, but an Incident Management Group will discuss this. Individual cases may be discussed with Occupational Health or Microbiology/Virology if required.

VISITORS   Visitors should be kept to a minimum. Children should not visit. Visitors should comply with infection control precautions.

PATIENT TRANSFER   Patient transfer should not occur unless clinically necessary, e.g. transfer to a specialist infectious diseases unit. The receiving ward/department must be informed in advance of the diagnosis.

MORE INFORMATION   Rabies is a serious, usually fatal infection, that affects the central nervous system to cause encephalitis. It is best managed in a specialist infectious diseases unit.

Most rabies infections occur in developing countries, particularly in South and South East Asia. Cases in the UK are rare and usually acquired in other countries. It is possible to acquire rabies in the UK from bats, which carry a rabies-like virus called European Bat Lyssavirus; terrestrial animals in the UK are rabies free.

There is no treatment for rabies, but vaccines are available that may be given either pre-exposure or post-exposure. Post-exposure prophylaxis (vaccination, with or without rabies immunoglobulin) can prevent rabies after a bite/exposure.

Travellers should always seek pre-travel advice about whether they need rabies vaccination and should minimise animal contact while abroad. If they receive an animal bite or scratch in a country where rabies is present, they should clean the wound thoroughly with soap and water and should seek medical advice immediately.

Up to date and country-specific information on rabies is available on the Health Protection Agency website www.hpa.org.uk or the NaTHNaC website www.nathnac.org.

Rash illness

There are numerous possible causes of a rash illness. It is important to reach a diagnosis as soon as possible, to guide clinical management and infection control.

Important infectious causes of rash illness include:

Vesicular (blistering) rash – chickenpox, shingles, hand, foot and mouth
Non-vesicular rash – scabies, meningococcal septicaemia, streptococcal infection, measles, rubella, parvovirus, cytomegalovirus, Epstein–Barr virus, human herpes virus 6 and 7, syphilis and some travel-associated infections

SPREAD BY   The route of spread depends on the causative organism; refer to the individual organism subsections in this chapter.

INFECTIOUS PERIOD   This depends on the causative organism. As a rough guide, most rash illnesses are infectious for a short time before the rash comes out and for the duration of the rash if untreated.

INFECTION CONTROL PRECAUTIONS

1	Isolation	Required
2	Hand washing	Required
3	Gloves	Required
4	Apron	Required
5	Mask	Not required
6	Eye protection	Not required

STAFF   Pregnant staff should not look after a patient with an undiagnosed rash. Some rash illnesses such as rubella, chickenpox and parvovirus have consequences in pregnancy. Discuss with Microbiology or Occupational Health if required.

VISITORS   Visitors should be kept to a minimum until a diagnosis is reached.

PATIENT TRANSFER   Patient transfer should be kept to a minimum. The area with the rash should be covered during transfer if possible. The receiving ward/department should be informed of the rash illness. Patients with a rash should not wait in communal areas such as waiting rooms.

MORE INFORMATION   Obtain a full history including travel history. Seek advice from Microbiology regarding appropriate investigations. A Dermatology review is always useful.

Respiratory syncytial virus (RSV)

Respiratory syncytial virus (RSV) is an RNA virus that is a common cause of respiratory tract infection, particularly in children.

SPREAD BY

- Direct contact (e.g. kissing a child with RSV).
- Indirect contact (e.g. touching a door knob contaminated with virus).
- Droplet spread (e.g. inhaling droplets of respiratory secretions immediately after a patient sneezes).

The virus is present in respiratory secretions of infected people and can remain viable for 4–7 hours on contaminated surfaces. Inhaling the virus or bringing it to the face (touching your own eyes, nose or mouth with contaminated hands) can spread infection. Good hand hygiene and environmental hygiene are paramount to prevent cross-infection.

INFECTIOUS PERIOD   The infectious period is usually 3–8 days. In practice, people are considered potentially infectious until their symptoms have resolved. Testing for clearance is not generally advisable, though may have a role in neonatal and paediatric critical care units.

Some infants and immunocompromised patients may be infectious for up to 4 weeks after RSV infection: speak to your Infection Prevention and Control Team before allowing them out of isolation.

IINFECTION CONTROL PRECAUTIONS

1	Isolation	Required – single room preferable, cohorting acceptable for laboratory confirmed cases
2	Hand washing	Required
3	Gloves	Required
4	Apron	Required
5	Mask	Not required
6	Eye protection	Not required

STAFF   No further precautions.

VISITORS   Visitors should be kept to a minimum and should perform hand hygiene before and after seeing the patient. They should be discouraged from visiting other patients or mixing with other relatives. They should not visit if they develop symptoms of respiratory tract infection.

PATIENT TRANSFER   Patient transfer should be kept to a minimum. The receiving ward/department should be informed of the diagnosis. If possible, a surgical mask should be worn during transfer.

CLEANING   Cleaning should be thorough (to remove environmental contamination) and should be increased during outbreaks. Once an RSV patient is discharged, the patient area must be thoroughly cleaned before it is put back into use.

COHORTING   Cohorting involves managing several patients with the same infection in a bay of a ward, rather than placing them separately in side rooms. It is commonly done for RSV infection on paediatric wards over the winter when several patients may be admitted each day with RSV infection. It is important to obtain laboratory results before cohorting, as other respiratory infections such as influenza or whooping cough could resemble RSV and should not be managed in the same bay. Staff in the cohort bay should be dedicated to that bay and should not work on other areas during the same shift.

MASKS   Masks are not generally required while caring for RSV patients, as droplet or aerosol transmission is uncommon.

MORE INFORMATION   In the United Kingdom, RSV infection peaks in the winter months (November–April) and is uncommon at other times of year. Many laboratories do not even test for RSV during the summer.

The spectrum of disease caused by RSV infection includes:

- mild respiratory tract infections with symptoms of cough, cold and fever;
- bronchiolitis – an infection of bronchioles (the small airways leading to the lung), which become inflamed and filled with mucus, causing cough, wheeze and shortness of breath;
- pneumonia;
- exacerbation of COPD.

RSV is the commonest cause of bronchiolitis in children under 1 year of age (70% of cases). Pneumonia is more likely to occur in immunocompromised patients, very premature infants or those with chronic lung disease.

Immunity against RSV is not lifelong and recurrent infections can occur.

Any patient attending a ward who has been in contact with a symptomatic case of RSV should be isolated as a precaution until the end of the incubation period (8 days).

Any patients who are exposed to RSV (e.g. nursed in a bay with a patient who subsequently develops RSV) should be managed as a contact: the index (symptomatic) case should be isolated, the other patients remain in the bay and the bay may need to be closed to admissions until the incubation period is up. This should be discussed with your Infection Prevention and Control Team.

RSV testing is available in most laboratories. Suitable samples are a nasopharyngeal aspirate or viral swabs of the nose and throat (check with your own laboratory). Results are usually available within a couple of hours for an EIA test (the commonest test). PCR testing is available in specialist centres and has a longer turnaround time.

No vaccine against RSV is available at present.

A monoclonal antibody against RSV (palivizumab) is available as prophylaxis against RSV for high-risk infants (premature or with cardiac or lung disease). Monthly injections are given during the RSV season (usually for 5 months).

Treatment is largely supportive. An antiviral drug called ribavirin is occasionally used in severe cases but its efficacy is limited and it has toxicities for patients and staff.

Rotavirus

Rotavirus is a virus that causes diarrhoea, vomiting and abdominal cramps. It is a common cause of viral gastroenteritis in children and can also affect adults.

SPREAD BY   Faecal–oral route: either by direct contact or via contaminated food or water. Transmission by environmental contamination can occur.

INFECTIOUS PERIOD   The incubation period is approximately 48 hours. The infectious period is from the onset of symptoms until 48 hours after the last episode of diarrhoea or vomiting. Symptoms usually last 3–8 days.

INFECTION CONTROL PRECAUTIONS

1	Isolation	Required
2	Hand washing	Required
3	Gloves	Required
4	Apron	Required
5	Mask	Not required
6	Eye protection	Not required

Patients with rotavirus should ideally be isolated in a side room. Patients with confirmed rotavirus infection may be cohorted together if insufficient side rooms are available.

STAFF   Any staff with rotavirus should be kept off work until 48 hours from the last episode of diarrhoea or vomiting.

VISITORS   Visitors should comply with the same precautions as staff and should be reminded not to eat or drink in the isolation room.

PATIENT TRANSFER   Patient transfer should be kept to a minimum while diarrhoea/vomiting symptoms persist. If the patient must be moved, inform the receiving ward/department of the diagnosis and ensure surfaces are wiped down with detergent after patient contact.

FURTHER INFORMATION   Rotavirus infections have a seasonal incidence, which peaks in the winter months.

There is no specific treatment for rotavirus.

Vaccination against rotavirus is used routinely in several countries and was added to the UK routine childhood immunisation schedule from autumn 2013.

Rubella (German measles)

Rubella is a vaccine-preventable disease of childhood, caused by the rubella virus. Its great significance is that rubella infection in pregnancy causes severe congenital problems known as congenital rubella syndrome. Rubella is a notifiable disease.

SPREAD BY   Droplet spread as virus is present in respiratory secretions and direct (vertical) transmission from mother to child during pregnancy.

INFECTIOUS PERIOD   The incubation period is 14–23 days (usually 16–18 days). The infectious period is from one week before the rash until 4 days after the onset of rash.

INFECTION CONTROL PRECAUTIONS

1	Isolation	Required
2	Hand washing	Required
3	Gloves	Required
4	Apron	Required
5	Mask	Not required
6	Eye protection	Not required

STAFF   Pregnant or non-immune staff should not care for a patient with suspected or confirmed rubella.

VISITORS   Pregnant women, or anyone who has not been vaccinated against rubella, should be discouraged from visiting.

PATIENT TRANSFER   Patient transfer should be avoided if possible during the infectious period. If transfer is necessary, it is advisable for the patient to wear a mask during transfer and the patient should not wait in a communal area such as a waiting room. The receiving ward/department must be informed of the diagnosis.

MORE INFORMATION   Rubella is usually a mild disease that causes headache, fever and a transient red rash, sometimes with swollen lymph glands around the ears (post-auricular) or back of the head (suboccipital). Adults may develop arthralgia, especially women. Sometimes infection is subclinical/asymptomatic.

It can be difficult to diagnose rubella clinically as its presentation is non-specific and resembles other viral infections. Clinical diagnosis should be confirmed using IgM and IgG serology. Oral fluid testing is arranged via the notification process.

Rubella in pregnancy is a serious issue. Congenital rubella leads to many problems including deafness, cataracts, learning difficulties, cardiac abnormalities and microcephaly. The risk of congenital rubella depends on the stage of pregnancy at which maternal infection occurs:

Less than 11 weeks	90%
11–16 weeks	20%
16–20 weeks	<10%, deafness only
>20 weeks	No increased risk

Any pregnant woman who may have been in contact with rubella should have rubella serology done, unless they have two previous positive tests showing pre-existing immunity to rubella. As a general principle, any pregnant woman with a rash illness or exposure to a rash illness should seek medical advice urgently.

Rubella vaccine is part of the MMR vaccine and is therefore within the UK childhood vaccination schedule. Healthcare workers should provide proof of vaccination to Occupational Health when they start work.

Salmonella

Salmonella infection is an important cause of diarrhoea. It is a notifiable disease. There are numerous species of *Salmonella*, most of which cause 'food poisoning' or gastroenteritis. This section deals with these common infections. Typhoid (caused by *Salmonella typhi*) and paratyphoid (caused by *Salmonella paratyphi*) are covered in their own subsections.

SPREAD BY   Consumption of contaminated food is the commonest cause of infection. *Salmonella* bacteria live in the gut of many farm animals and may be present in meat (especially poultry), eggs and unpasteurised milk. These foods may contaminate other foods (e.g. if raw and cooked foods are stored together in a fridge). Other foods such as fruit and vegetables may rarely be contaminated via manure in the soil or sewage in the water. Faecal–oral spread from person to person may occur if there are lapses in hygiene such as inadequate hand hygiene after going to the toilet or before and after handling food. Pet reptiles frequently carry *Salmonella* and can pass infection to their handlers.

INFECTIOUS PERIOD   The incubation period is 12 hours to 3 days. Symptoms last for 4 to 7 days. Cases are considered infectious until 48 hours after the symptoms have stopped, although carriage may continue for longer periods. Food handlers and other people at high risk of transmitting disease may need stool screening for clearance – discuss with Public Health.

INFECTION CONTROL PRECAUTIONS

1	**Isolation**	Required
2	**Hand washing**	Required
3	**Gloves**	Required
4	**Apron**	Required
5	**Mask**	Not required
6	**Eye protection**	Not required

STAFF   Staff should ensure there is no uncovered food near the patient and should not eat in clinical areas.

VISITORS   Visitors should not eat or drink while visiting the patient and must wash their hands before and after the visit.

PATIENT TRANSFER   The receiving ward/department should be informed of the diagnosis.

MORE INFORMATION   Symptoms of *Salmonella* infection include diarrhoea, stomach cramps and sometimes vomiting and fever. Infection is usually self-limiting, i.e. most people get better without antibiotics. *Salmonella* infection can be more serious in the very young, elderly or immunosuppressed.

Scabies (*Sarcoptes scabiei* var. *hominis*)

There are two types of scabies infestation: classical and crusted. The same mite causes both, but in crusted scabies there are many more mites. Crusted scabies is sometimes referred to as 'Norwegian' or 'atypical' scabies. Both types are discussed below – first classical, then crusted.

Scabies (both crusted and classical) is difficult to diagnose. If you suspect your patient has scabies you should ask for an urgent dermatological review and adopt the infection control precautions set out below until scabies has been either ruled out or treated.

Classical scabies

Classical scabies is the type most commonly seen.

SPREAD BY   Scabies mites cannot jump or fly; they have to crawl from one person to another. Therefore direct skin-to-skin contact with an infested person for a prolonged period of time is required for transmission to occur. Provision of close personal care could lead to transmission but brief contact, such as a handshake, would not.

INFECTIOUS PERIOD   Classical scabies requires two applications of treatment, one week apart; an infested person remains infectious until 24 hours after the first treatment has been applied.

INFECTION CONTROL PRECAUTIONS

1	Isolation	Required
2	Hand washing	Required
3	Gloves	Required
4	Apron	A long-sleeved gown should be worn in order to cover the arms fully during patient contact
5	Mask	Not required
6	Eye protection	Not required

STAFF   Staff are at risk of scabies infestation during patient contact and should wear gloves and gowns for all contact with suspected/confirmed scabies.

VISITORS   Visitors should adopt the same precautions as staff.

PATIENT TRANSFER   Transfer should be avoided until 24 hours after application of the first treatment. If transfer is absolutely necessary it is essential that staff in the receiving ward/department are informed of the patient's scabies infestation prior to transfer, in order to ensure that they have access to gowns and gloves.

TREATMENT OF CLASSICAL SCABIES   Permethrin is the treatment of choice but Malathion can be used if Permethrin is not suitable. Permethrin cream should be applied all over the body including the scalp, genitals, behind the ears and under the nails and left on for 8–12 hours (overnight is often a good option). If the cream has to be washed off any area within the 8–12 hour period it should be reapplied to that area. Two applications of Permethrin, one week apart, are required.

After treatment, bedding and clothing should be washed at 60°C. If washing is not possible the items should be placed in a bag and left for three days before being laundered or reused to allow the mites to die.

Crusted scabies

Crusted scabies is a more severe form of scabies where thousands or even millions of scabies mites are present. It is less common than classical scabies and tends to occur in those who are immunocompromised, very elderly or with neurological disorders.

SPREAD BY   Crusted scabies is highly infectious; the proliferation of mites means that there may be many thousands on the patient's skin, clothing and bedding. Mites are dispersed into the air during personal care, bedmaking, etc., contaminating the environment by airborne spread. As such all contact with the patient and their environment can lead to transmission.

INFECTIOUS PERIOD   Crusted scabies requires multiple treatments and as such it is advisable to continue isolation precautions for 10 days after treatment commences.

INFECTION CONTROL PRECAUTIONS

1	Isolation	Required
2	Hand washing	Required
3	Gloves	Required
4	Apron	A long-sleeved gown should be worn in order to cover the arms fully during patient contact
5	Mask	Not required
6	Eye protection	Not required

STAFF   Staff are at risk of infestation from crusted scabies during contact with the patient and their surroundings and should wear gloves and gowns for all contact.

VISITORS   Visitors should adopt the same precautions as staff.

PATIENT TRANSFER   Transfer should be avoided until completion of treatment. If transfer is absolutely necessary it is essential that staff in the receiving ward/department are informed of the patient's scabies infestation prior to transfer, in order to ensure that they have access to gowns and gloves.

TREATMENT   Permethrin is the treatment of choice but Malathion can be used if Permethrin is not suitable. Permethrin cream should be applied all over the body including the scalp, genitals, behind the ears and under the nails and left on for 8–12 hours (overnight is often a good option). If the cream has to be washed off any area within the 8–12 hour period it should be reapplied to that area. Multiple applications of Permethrin may be required to treat crusted scabies and oral Ivermectin may be added.

After treatment, bedding and clothing should be washed at 60°C. If washing is not possible the items should be placed in a bag and left for three days before being laundered or reused to allow the mites to die. The patient's environment will require thorough cleaning, including vacuuming of soft furnishings and upholstery, to remove the mites.

OUTBREAK MANAGEMENT   Before commencing any treatment regime it is important to talk to the microbiologist and Infection Control Team. One case of scabies in a healthcare setting will require treatment of that case alone, whereas two or more cases in a healthcare setting will require contact tracing and prophylactic treatment for (potential) patients, and a number of staff who will require input from the Occupational Health Team

Scarlet fever (scarletina)

Scarlet fever is a childhood disease caused by infection with Group A streptococcus. The bacteria usually infect the throat first (pharyngitis) and then produce a toxin that affects the skin to cause a characteristic rash. Scarlet fever is a notifiable disease.

SPREAD BY   The bacteria are present in the throat, saliva and nasal mucus of an infected person. Infection may be spread by:

- Direct person-to-person contact.
- Indirect contact, e.g. shared drinking glasses or eating utensils.
- Droplet spread, i.e. inhaling airborne droplets if the patient coughs or sneezes near you.

INFECTIOUS PERIOD   The incubation period is 2–5 days. The infectious period is for the duration of the illness if untreated (about a week) or until 24 hours of appropriate antibiotics have been given.

INFECTION CONTROL PRECAUTIONS

1	Isolation	Required
2	Hand washing	Required
3	Gloves	Required
4	Apron	Required
5	Mask	Not required
6	Eye protection	Not required

STAFF   No further precautions.

VISITORS   No further precautions.

PATIENT TRANSFER   Patient transfer should be kept to a minimum for the first 24 hours of treatment. The receiving ward/department must be informed of the diagnosis.

MORE INFORMATION   Clinical features are a sore throat initially, followed 1–2 days later by a widespread rash, which starts on the face but spares the lips (circumoral pallor) and then spreads to the trunk and limbs but spares the palms and soles. The rash is blanching and erythematous, and it feels like sandpaper because the skin around the hair follicles rises up. The tongue has a characteristic 'strawberry tongue' appearance. The rash desquamates (peels off) later in the illness. Other symptoms include fever, flushed cheeks, headache, nausea and vomiting.

Investigations should include a throat swab and serum for ASOT.

Treatment is with penicillin for 10 days.

Most people make a full recovery although rare complications include glomerulonephritis and rheumatic fever.

Serratia

Serratia is a Gram-negative rod (bacterium) found in the environment and in the gut. It mainly causes healthcare-associated infections such as hospital acquired/ventilator-associated pneumonia, urinary tract infection, wound infection and bacteremia.

SPREAD BY   Direct spread, e.g. on the hands of staff, or indirect spread, e.g. via contaminated equipment (particularly equipment that has a water reservoir) or contaminated feeds.

INFECTIOUS PERIOD   Indefinite, as gut carriage (colonisation) occurs and is difficult to eradicate.

INFECTION CONTROL PRECAUTIONS

1	**Isolation**	Not required
2	**Hand washing**	Required
3	**Gloves**	Not required
4	**Apron**	Not required
5	**Mask**	Not required
6	**Eye protection**	Not required

STAFF   No further restrictions.

VISITORS   No restrictions.

PATIENT TRANSFER   No restrictions.

MORE INFORMATION   Outbreaks of *Serratia* have been seen on neonatal ICUs, presenting with bacteremia, meningitis or eye infections. Serratia can be resistant to several classes of antibiotic such as cephalosporins and quinolones.

Shigella

Shigella infection is an important cause of infective diarrhoea and dysentery (diarrhoea with blood and mucus). It is a notifiable disease.

SPREAD BY   Faecal–oral spread may occur via direct contact with cases, or by consumption of contaminated water or food, or by indirect contact (e.g. contaminated surfaces). Outbreaks of *S. sonnei* infection have been seen in schools and nurseries in the UK, probably due to poor hand hygiene and toilet hygiene. Infection may also be sexually transmitted, mainly among men who have sex with men.

INFECTIOUS PERIOD   *Shigella* is highly infectious, with ingestion of as few as 10 organisms being sufficient to cause infection. The incubation period is 12 hours to 4 days. Cases remain infectious for as long as the organism is excreted in the stool, which is 2–4 weeks on average.

INFECTION CONTROL PROCEDURES

1	Isolation	Required
2	Hand washing	Required
3	Gloves	Required
4	Apron	Required
5	Mask	Not required
6	Eye protection	Not required

STAFF   Staff should ensure that there is no uncovered food near the patient and should not eat in clinical areas – this is standard good practice but is particularly important with *Shigella* as it is so infectious.

VISITORS   Visitors should not eat or drink while visiting the patient and must wash their hands before and after the visit.

PATIENT TRANSFER   The receiving ward/department should be informed of the diagnosis.

MORE INFORMATION   There are four species of *Shigella* that cause infection: *Shigella sonnei* is endemic in the UK, and the other species (*Shigella dysenteriae*, *Shigella boydii* and *Shigella flexneri*) are usually travel-associated.

Shigella can produce a toxin known as Shiga toxin, which is associated with cell damage and haemolytic uraemic syndrome (an uncommon complication of shigellosis).

Shigella survives well in the environment for up to 20 days.

Shingles (herpes zoster)

Caused by the varicella zoster virus (VZV).

SPREAD BY   Shingles cannot be caught. It is a reactivation of the varicella zoster virus that has lain dormant in the nerve ganglia following chicken pox infection earlier in life. The liquid in the shingles blisters (vesicles) is infected with VZV and direct contact with the fluid can result in chicken pox infection in people who are not immune to chicken pox.

Shingles is not spread by respiratory droplets and is much less infectious than chicken pox. However, in the healthcare setting more cases of chickenpox in staff are caused by contact with shingles because the rash is often not recognised as such for several days. During this period, staff with no immunity to chickenpox may be exposed.

Immunocompromised patients may develop a more widespread shingles rash than immunocompetent patients and as such are more infectious.

INFECTIOUS PERIOD   From the onset of the rash until all blisters have crusted over.

INFECTION CONTROL PRECAUTIONS

1	**Isolation**	Required
2	**Hand washing**	Required
3	**Gloves**	Required
4	**Apron**	Required
5	**Mask**	Required if there is a risk of splash of vesicle fluid
6	**Eye protection**	Required if there is a risk of splash of vesicle fluid

STAFF

- Healthcare workers (HCWs) caring for patients with shingles must be certain that they have had chickenpox in the past or otherwise should have been vaccinated against varicella. If in doubt contact Occupational Health to arrange to have blood tested for VZV IgG.
- Pregnant HCWs with no immunity or uncertain immunity to chickenpox must avoid contact with shingles and have blood taken to determine their immune status.
- HCWs suspected of having shingles must report to Occupational Health. If the lesions are covered by clothing and not exposed then the staff member can continue to work providing they feel well enough to do so and do not work in a high-risk area with immunocompromised or vulnerable patients.
- HCWs should have their immunity to chickenpox tested by Occupational Health at the time of joining the organisation. A vaccine is available for non-immune staff via Occupational Health.

VISITORS   Inform visitors of the infection and only allow those with a past history of/ known immunity to chickenpox to visit.

PATIENT TRANSFER   Only move the patient if absolutely necessary. Cover the affected area if possible and inform the receiving area of their shingles status prior to transfer.

MORE INFORMATION   The shingles rash is usually preceded by pain in the area where the rash develops, typically the chest or face, and the rash affects only one side of the body.

The risk of shingles is increased with HIV infection, immunosuppression and old age. It is possible but rare to have shingles more than once.

Shingles can cause a condition called post-herpetic neuralgia, where the sufferer experiences pain long after the rash has cleared up.

Non-immune infants exposed to shingles (other than from their mother) in the first seven days of life, or whilst in intensive/special care, and pregnant women are at greater risk of infection if the exposure is to uncovered shingles lesions or to an immunocompromised person with shingles. Discuss any such cases with Microbiology, as they may require varicella zoster immunoglobulin (VZIG).

Staphylococcus aureus

This bacterium colonises up to a third of the population, but is also an important pathogen.

SPREAD BY   Many *S. aureus* infections are autoinfections, i.e. the patient's own colonising flora causes an infection. This is particularly likely if there is a break in the skin such as minor trauma or a leg ulcer. *S. aureus* may also be transmitted by direct person-to-person contact, indirect contact, e.g. via a dirty or dusty equipment, or airborne spread, e.g. from clouds of staphylococci dispersed during bedmaking.

INFECTIOUS PERIOD   The infectious period is difficult to define because so many people are colonised long term with *S. aureus*. For the purpose of infection control, a patient with an SSTI is usually regarded as potentially infectious until they have completed 24 hours on appropriate antibiotics. However, *S. aureus* is so common that enhanced precautions are not generally taken unless it is shown to be a particularly resistant strain (such as MRSA) or virulent strain (such as PVL).

INFECTION CONTROL PRECAUTIONS

1	**Isolation**	Not required
2	**Hand washing**	Required
3	**Gloves**	Not required
4	**Apron**	Not required
5	**Mask**	Not required
6	**Eye protection**	Not required

STAFF   No further precautions.

VISITORS   No further precautions.

PATIENT TRANSFER   The infected area should be covered with an impermeable dressing if possible. Otherwise no restrictions.

MORE INFORMATION   20–30% of people carry *S. aureus* in the nose (anterior nares). It can cause a range of infections including:

- skin and soft tissue infections (SSTI), such as impetigo, cellulitis, paronychia, abscesses
- conjunctivitis
- wound and IV line infections
- pneumonia
- deep-seated infections such as osteomyelitis, septic arthritis, endocarditis
- toxic shock syndrome
- bacteremia.

Staphylococcus aureus can be diagnosed by microscopy and culture. Treatment requires drainage of pus and removal of foreign bodies where possible, plus antibiotics if clinically necessary.

Stenotrophomonas

Stenotrophomonas maltophilia is an environmental bacterium that may be found in hospitals and that can cause infections including respiratory tract infections, urinary tract infections, surgical site infections and bacteremia. It is intrinsically resistant to many antibiotics. Infections occur mainly in patients who are immunocompromised, have had a prolonged hospital stay, have had broad-spectrum antibiotics (particularly meropenem) or have been ventilated.

SPREAD BY   Direct contact: transfer on hands from an environmental source. Indirect contact: transfer from equipment/environment.

INFECTIOUS PERIOD   *Stenotrophomonas* is not readily transferred between patients provided standard principles of infection control are followed, but theoretically a patient may remain colonised and potentially infectious for months or years.

INFECTION CONTROL PRECAUTIONS   In a community setting or in a general ward, standard principles of infection control are adequate. In high-dependency areas such as ITU, isolation may be required.

1	Isolation	Not usually required (seek advice if patient on ITU/HDU)
2	Hand washing	Required
3	Gloves	Not required
4	Apron	Not required
5	Mask	Not required
6	Eye protection	Not required

STAFF   No additional precautions required.

VISITORS   No restrictions.

PATIENT TRANSFER   No restrictions.

MORE INFORMATION   *Stenotrophomonas* does not commonly cause clinical infections. It can usually be treated with co-trimoxazole if antibiotics are required.

Frequent detection of *Stenotrophomonas* in patient samples from a ward may indicate overuse of carbapenem antibiotics (such as meropenem) and may require increased antibiotic stewardship.

Toxoplasmosis

A zoonotic (animal-transmitted) infection caused by infection with the parasite *Toxoplasma gondii*. Infection is more serious in pregnant women and immunocompromised patients.

SPREAD BY   Contact with cat faeces, e.g. cleaning out cat litter trays. Ingesting water, food or soil contaminated with the faeces of infected animals, e.g. unwashed salad. Eating undercooked meat containing cysts. Vertical transmission from mother to foetus. Receiving an organ transplant from a donor with acute or latent toxoplasmosis.

Direct person-to-person transmission does not occur, except from mother to foetus. See below for an explanation of the life-cycle and how transmission occurs.

INFECTIOUS PERIOD   The incubation period is 5–20 days for acute infection. Reactivation of infection can occur years after the original exposure.

There is no recognised infectious period because person-to-person transmission does not occur.

INFECTION CONTROL PRECAUTIONS

1	**Isolation**	Not required
2	**Hand washing**	Required
3	**Gloves**	Not required
4	**Apron**	Not required
5	**Mask**	Not required
6	**Eye protection**	Not required

STAFF   No further precautions.

VISITORS   No further precautions.

PATIENT TRANSFER   No restrictions.

MORE INFORMATION   *Toxoplasma gondii* infects all mammal and bird species worldwide and it is estimated that up to one billion people worldwide have been exposed.

The life-cycle is complicated, but essentially cats are the main 'definitive' host in which the parasite completes its life-cycle. An infected cat sheds the parasite as cysts in its stool, which can subsequently infect people or other mammals who ingest them. Once *Toxoplasma* has entered the body, it causes a primary infection and then disseminates via the bloodstream to form tissue cysts, which lie latent for years but which can reactivate if you become immunocompromised.

The primary infection is often asymptomatic but can cause an illness resembling glandular fever with fever, generalised lymphadenopathy, headache and myalgia.

Other clinical scenarios are: ocular infection (usually due to reactivation of the disease); toxoplasmosis in the immunocompromised, which is usually due to reactivation and often affects the central nervous system; and congenital toxoplasmosis.

Pregnant women should avoid exposure to toxoplasmosis by modifying their diet and avoiding contact with cat faeces. Congenital toxoplasmosis can cause foetal abnormalities or death – the effect depends upon the gestation at the time of infection. Any pregnant woman who is concerned about toxoplasmosis should seek medical advice.

Treatment for toxoplasmosis is available but is not generally required in immunocompetent, non-pregnant patients. In other cases, specialist advice should be sought.

No vaccine is available.

Tuberculosis (TB)

Infection is caused by the bacterium *Mycobacterium tuberculosis*. Respiratory TB is the commonest presentation, but TB can infect other body sites. Only respiratory TB is infectious. TB is a notifiable disease.

SPREAD BY   Droplet spread: patients with respiratory TB may expel droplets containing infectious TB bacteria into the air when they cough or sneeze. If these droplets are inhaled they can cause TB infection. Prolonged or close exposure is generally required to catch TB.

INFECTIOUS PERIOD   The incubation period is variable: approximately 4–12 weeks from exposure to primary infection, though the disease may reactivate months or years later.
   A patient with infectious respiratory TB will remain infectious indefinitely if untreated. Patients are usually no longer infectious once they have completed 2 weeks of appropriate therapy.

INFECTION CONTROL PRECAUTIONS   Patients with known or suspected TB should not be admitted to hospital unless necessary. Patients with respiratory TB should always be isolated in a side room pending laboratory results, and should always be separated from immunocompromised patients (HIV, transplant, oncology, etc.), either by admission to a single room on a separate ward or in a negative-pressure room on the same ward. NICE guidance states that mask, gown and isolation precautions are not required unless the patient has multidrug-resistant TB (MDR-TB) or is undergoing an aerosol-generating procedure. This is a change from previous practice and some hospitals still recommend apron, gloves and FFP3 masks. Check your local policy.

1	Isolation	Smear-positive patients – required until 2 weeks treatment completed
		Smear-negative or non-respiratory disease – not required
		Children – required*
		Drug-resistant TB – requires negative pressure isolation room
2	Hand washing	Required
3	Gloves	Not required unless handling body fluids
4	Apron	Not required unless handling body fluids
5	Mask	FFP3 mask required for MDR TB or aerosol-generating procedures
6	Eye protection	Not required

*Children with TB should be isolated until the source case has been identified, regardless of AFB smear results. This is because the source case is likely to be a relative who visits the ward. These visitors should only visit the isolation room and then leave – they should not spend time in communal areas until they have been screened and infection excluded.

Patients should perform respiratory hygiene (Chapter 2). Aerosol-generating procedures such as bronchoscopy should be carried out in a negative pressure room or bronchoscopy suite. Staff should wear gowns, gloves and FFP3 masks.

STAFF   The number of staff caring for infectious TB patients should be kept to a reasonable minimum, without compromising patient care. Staff who are likely to work with TB patients should be fit tested for FFP3 mask use. Staff who work with patient or clinical materials should complete a health check including TB assessment when they start in the job. This includes a history/health questionnaire and BCG scar check. Mantoux skin testing or interferon-gamma testing may be offered if appropriate.

VISITORS   Visitors should be restricted to immediate family and those who have already been in close contact with the patient before diagnosis. Visitors are discouraged from bringing in babies and children.

PATIENT TRANSFER   Patient transfer should be kept to a minimum until the patient has completed 2 weeks of treatment. Inpatients with smear-positive respiratory TB should wear a surgical mask whenever they leave their room until they have had 2 weeks of treatment. The receiving ward/department must be informed of the diagnosis. Patients should not wait in communal areas such as waiting rooms.

LINEN AND LAUNDRY   Linen and laundry should go into a red linen bag.

MORE INFORMATION   Tuberculosis infection rates are increasing, both in the UK and worldwide. There are approximately 9000 cases in the UK each year, most of which occur in cities (particularly in London).

Respiratory tuberculosis is active TB affecting any of the following: lungs, pleural cavity, medastinal lymph nodes, larynx. Symptoms may include a cough lasting longer than 3 weeks, fatigue, weight loss, night sweats, dyspnoea, haemoptysis or chest pain. Some patients are asymptomatic. Chest X ray is abnormal.

Non-respiratory tuberculosis may affect various body sites to cause bone and joint infection, meningitis, lymphadenitis, pericarditis, disseminated (miliary) TB, genitourinary TB or gastrointestinal TB.

HIV patients are at increased risk of symptomatic TB infection.

DIAGNOSIS OF TB   Diagnosis of TB is usually by chest X-ray and three sputum samples sent on consecutive days for acid-fast bacilli (AFB) investigation. Other samples such as bronchial washings or gastric washings in children (who swallow sputum instead of coughing it up) are acceptable. For non-respiratory TB, pus or tissue may be sent in a universal container (not formalin).

A 'smear' of the sputum is examined under a microscope for AFBs. Results are used to establish whether the patient is likely to be infectious to others: smear-positive patients are infectious; smear-negative patients where the culture result is not yet known are potentially infectious but low risk for transmission; and patients who are sputum smear and culture-negative, or who have non-respiratory TB, are non-infectious. Patients whose bronchial washings are smear-positive are not regarded as infectious unless their sputum is also smear-positive or becomes so after bronchoscopy.

PCR and/or culture are required for full identification and sensitivity testing of AFBs. Other tests for TB include interferon-gamma testing (a blood test for latent TB) and Mantoux testing (a skin test used to diagnose latent TB).

MANAGEMENT   The respiratory medical team and a specialist TB nurse should always be involved in the management of TB. They oversee diagnosis, treatment and contact tracing. Treatment requires at least 6 months of combination antibiotics with close follow-up.

Contact tracing in the hospital setting is only required if there was a delay in isolating the patient. Other patients are considered at risk of infection if they have spent more than 8 hours in the same bay as an inpatient with sputum smear-positive TB who had a cough.

DRUG RESISTANCE   Drug-resistant strains are more difficult to treat and have worse outcomes. Patients with suspected MDR TB must be managed in a negative pressure room and preferably transferred to a specialist unit. Staff and visitors should wear FFP3 masks.

Mono-resistant = resistant to one drug; poly-resistant = resistant to >1 drug (but not MDR); multidrug resistant (MDR) = resistant to at least rifampicin and isoniazid; extensively drug resistant (XDR) = resistant to rifampicin, isoniazid, a quinolone and an injectable agent.

Typhoid

A systemic infection with pronounced gastrointestinal symptoms, caused by infection with *Salmonella typhi* (also known as *Salmonella enterica* serovar typhi). Typhoid is a notifiable disease.

SPREAD BY   The infection is present in the stools and sometimes in the blood and urine of an infected person. The commonest mode of spread is faecal–oral, usually through contaminated water (mainly in the developing world) or by contamination of food. Direct person-to-person faecal–oral transmission can occur in poor hygiene conditions or in men who have sex with men.

Household transmission of infection may occur, probably through lapses in food hygiene. Most cases in the UK are acquired abroad.

INFECTIOUS PERIOD   The incubation period is 7–14 days. Patients may remain infectious for several weeks after infection. Approximately 5% of cases become chronic carriers who continue to shed bacteria in the stool indefinitely.

INFECTION CONTROL PRECAUTIONS

1	**Isolation**	Required
2	**Hand washing**	Required
3	**Gloves**	Required
4	**Apron**	Required
5	**Mask**	Not required unless there is a significant risk of splashing to the face
6	**Eye protection**	Not required

STAFF   No additional precautions.

VISITORS   Visitors should be reminded not to eat or drink in the patient's room. They should wear PPE as above and should wash their hands when leaving the isolation room.

PATIENT TRANSFER   Patient transfer should only occur if necessary and the receiving ward/department must be informed of the diagnosis.

MORE INFORMATION   Infection with typhoid or paratyphoid is known as enteric fever. Clinical features of typhoid include fever of 39–40 °C, myalgia, abdominal pain and severe headache. Some patients have a rash on the trunk known as 'rose spots'. Diarrhoea is present in less than half of patients. Typhoid is a serious illness, with 20% mortality if untreated due to intestinal perforation or haemorrhage. Even when treated it may take several days to respond, with resolution of fever over 2–5 days and convalescence over several weeks.

The choice of antibiotic depends on sensitivity test results, as resistance is becoming increasingly common. The drug of choice is ciprofloxacin but alternatives include ceftriaxone and azithromycin.

Diagnosis is usually by stool sample, but blood or urine culture may also be positive. Serology is rarely useful.

Typhoid patients who are at high risk of passing it on, such as food handlers, should be screened for clearance by stool sample analysis on the advice of public or environmental health. The famous 'Typhoid Mary' was a cook and typhoid carrier in the early twentieth century who caused numerous outbreaks of typhoid!

Preventative measures include pre-travel hygiene advice and vaccination. Vaccination is not recommended for contacts of cases as it has not been shown to be effective in these circumstances.

Viral haemorrhagic fevers (VHFs)

Viral haemorrhagic fevers (VHFs) are imported infections caused by a range of viruses. VHF infection is uncommon but is important because it is difficult to diagnose, has a high case-fatality rate with no effective treatment and it can spread rapidly within the hospital setting unless correct precautions are taken. All units admitting returning travellers should have policies in place to risk assess and identify possible cases. Standard principles of infection control should be used while the assessment is carried out. Following the assessment, the patient is categorised as one of the following: highly unlikely to have VHF, possibility of VHF, high possibility of VHF or confirmed VHF. Further management, including the level of infection control precautions, depends on the outcome of the risk assessment. Always inform the Infection Prevention and Control Team and a consultant microbiologist of any suspected case of VHF. VHF is a notifiable disease: notify high possibility/confirmed cases urgently.

SPREAD BY

- Direct contact – if blood or body fluids come into contact with broken skin or mucous membranes.
- Indirect contact – with an environment contaminated with splashes or droplets of blood or body fluids.

INFECTIOUS PERIOD   The incubation period ranges from 3 to 21 days. The patient is considered potentially infectious until an alternative diagnosis is confirmed or until there has been a negative VHF screen and the patient has been afebrile for 24 hours. If VHF is the confirmed diagnosis, the patient is considered infectious for an indefinite period (seek expert guidance).

INFECTION CONTROL PRECAUTIONS
For patient highly unlikely to have VHF (no risk/ minimal risk)

1	Isolation	Not required
2	Hand washing	Required
3	Gloves	Required
4	Apron	Required
5	Mask	Not required
6	Eye protection	Not required

If possibility of VHF

1	Isolation	Required. Should have dedicated en suite facilities or dedicated commode
2	Hand washing	Required
3	Gloves	Required
4	Apron	Required
5	Mask	Not generally required, but if patient is bruising or bleeding wear a fluid-repellent surgical facemask for routine care and FFP3 mask for aerosol- or splash-generating procedures
6	Eye protection	Not generally required, but disposable visor recommended if patient is bruising or bleeding

For high possibility of VHF in a stable patient

1	**Isolation**	Required. Should have dedicated en suite facilities or dedicated commode
2	**Hand washing**	Required
3	**Gloves**	Required
4	**Apron**	Required
5	**Mask**	Required: fluid-repellent surgical mask generally adequate, FFP3 mask for aerosol- or splash-generating procedures
6	**Eye protection**	Required – disposable visor

For high possibility of VHF in patient with bruising, bleeding or uncontrolled diarrhoea/vomiting

1	**Isolation**	Required. Should have dedicated en suite facilities or dedicated commode
2	**Hand washing**	Required
3	**Gloves**	Double gloves required
4	**Apron**	Fluid-repellent disposable gown required
5	**Mask**	FFP3 mask required
6	**Eye protection**	Disposable visor required

EQUIPMENT   Equipment used in high-possibility/confirmed cases of VHF should be single use and disposable.

STAFF   If there is a high possibility of VHF, or a confirmed case, the number of staff caring for the patient should be restricted to essential staff only and a record of these staff should be kept. Remember to inform the laboratory of a suspected case of VHF so that laboratory staff can take appropriate precautions when handling specimens.

VISITORS   Visitors should not be allowed if there is a high possibility or confirmed case of VHF.

PATIENT TRANSFER   Patient transfer should not take place unless absolutely essential for medical reasons. The receiving department should be informed in advance of the possibility of VHF. The Infection Prevention and Control Team should also be informed of any planned patient movement.

MORE INFORMATION   Symptoms include fever, sore throat, headache, muscle or joint pain, diarrhoea and vomiting. Obvious bleeding occurs at a late stage of the illness. Cases of VHF are rare in the United Kingdom and are always imported from other countries. Any patient with high-possibility VHF, or with possible VHF with bruising or bleeding, must be discussed with an infectious disease unit. Any patient with confirmed VHF must be transferred to a high-security infectious disease unit. Management of a confirmed VHF case is a highly specialist subject and is not within the scope of this book.

Whooping cough

Whooping cough is a respiratory infection caused by the bacterium *Bordetella pertussis*. Whooping cough is a notifiable disease.

SPREAD BY   Close direct contact with an infected person, by droplet spread. It is highly contagious – up to 90% of susceptible household contacts will develop the disease.

INFECTIOUS PERIOD   The incubation period is usually 7–10 days (rarely it can be up to 21 days). The infectious period is up to 3 weeks after the onset of symptoms. Beyond 3 weeks, risk of transmission of infection is minimal, even if the cough persists.

INFECTIOUS CONTROL PRECAUTIONS

1	Isolation	Required
2	Hand washing	Required
3	Gloves	Required
4	Apron	Required
5	Mask	Required
6	Eye protection	Not required

The risk of transmission is minimal after 3 weeks of illness, but in a few cases (up to 20%) infectivity can persist for up to 6 weeks. Therefore the above infection control precautions should be taken in all hospitalised cases. Discuss with your Infection Prevention and Control Team if required.

STAFF   All staff looking after a patient with whooping cough should have had a full course of whooping cough vaccination. If vaccination history is incomplete or unknown, arrange for other staff to care for the patient and discuss with Occupational Health.

VISITORS   Visitors should be kept to a minimum number and should be limited to adults with a history of vaccination against whooping cough. Children under the age of 1 year should not visit under any circumstances. Visitors should comply with all above precautions.

PATIENT TRANSFER   Patient transfer should be kept to a minimum. The patient should wear a mask during transfer. The receiving ward/department should be informed in advance of the diagnosis.

MORE INFORMATION   Whooping cough may occur at any age. Young infants are the most at risk because they are not yet vaccinated and because infection at this age can cause severe illness with breathing difficulties.

Epidemics of whooping cough occur every 3 to 4 years, and the highest number of cases is usually in July–September annually.

Whooping cough is a vaccine-preventable disease. In the UK it is given as part of the routine childhood immunisation programme and is also given to high-risk groups as needed, e.g. to pregnant women during the 2012–2013 national outbreak. Immunity wanes over time and it is possible to catch whooping cough even if you have previously had the illness or a course of vaccinations.

The illness begins with coryzal symptoms and progresses to a dry cough, which may occur in paroxysms (outbursts of coughing) and may end with vomiting or with an intake of air, which makes a 'whooping' sound. The cough may go on for weeks or months.

Whooping cough is treated with antibiotics (usually erythromycin, clarithromycin or azithromycin) within the first 3 weeks of symptoms. Treatment is not necessary later in the course of the illness. Treatment duration used to be 14 days but has now been reduced to 7 days (3 days if taking azithromycin). Unvaccinated/partially vaccinated cases up to 10 years of age should complete their course of primary immunisation and booster vaccine once they have recovered from their acute illness.

Contacts of cases may be offered antibiotic prophylaxis and/or vaccination if identified promptly.

Laboratory confirmation is possible by culture or PCR of pernasal swab or nasopharyngeal aspirate, or by serology. Discuss with your microbiologist or Health Protection Unit to ascertain the most appropriate test.

5 Glossary

Adhesins Microbial factors that enable bacteria to adhere to cells.

Aerosol-generating procedure A procedure that can create an aerosol of the patient's secretions, e.g. oro/nasopharyngeal suctioning, positive pressure ventilation, cardiopulmonary resuscitation, chest physiotherapy, bronchoscopy, creating droplets small and light enough to become airborne, increasing the possibility for transmission of infection to occur.

Alcohol handrub An alcohol-based liquid, foam or gel for use on the hands to disinfect the skin.

Alert organisms Organisms that can cause outbreaks of infection that are difficult to treat due to antibiotic resistance.

Antibiogram A report that shows which of the antibiotics that are routinely tested will inhibit the growth of or kill the infectious agents they are tested on. Used to help make decisions about which antibiotics to use.

Asepsis The freedom from contamination by pathogenic organisms.

Aseptic technique A procedure or practice used to avoid introducing bacteria to a susceptible site, e.g. wound care, intravenous infusion management, insertion of invasive devices.

Augmented care unit Clinical areas with a high level of intervention, such as intensive therapy, high dependency and neonatal care units.

Auto-infection When microorganisms already present on the body cause an infection.

Bacteraemia The presence of an infectious agent in the blood.

Bactericidal Kills bacteria.

Bacteriostatic Inhibits bacterial growth but does not kill bacteria.

Bay A hospital room where more than one inpatient can stay that may have between two and six beds.

Bloodborne virus Viruses that are carried in the bloodstream, e.g. HIV, hepatitis B, hepatitis C.

Cadaver Dead body.

Case A person with clinical signs of infection (see below).

CE mark A visible sign that the manufacturer of the product is declaring conformity with all of the Directives relating to that product.

Cleaning The complete removal of soil from a medical device employing manual or automated processes.

Clinical signs of infection Typically, these are pyrexia, diarrhoea, an unexplained rash, localised redness, heat, pain, swelling and loss of function at the site. Other signs include increased exudate or slowness to heal or show any signs of improvement in a wound. If the patent has a urinary tract infection they may have dysuria, confusion, frequency of micturition. It is essential to look for clinical signs of infection when managing patients and not to focus solely on microbiological reports.

Rapid Infection Control Nursing, First Edition. Shona Ross and Sarah Furrows.
© 2014 John Wiley & Sons, Ltd. Published 2014 by John Wiley & Sons, Ltd.

Co-infection   When a person is infected with more than one infective agent at the same time.

Cohort   A group.

Cohorting   Nursing patients grouped together because they either have the same infection or have been exposed to the same type of infection.

Coliforms   Gram-negative bacilli of the *Enterobacteriaceae* spp. found in the intestines of humans and animals. Many coliforms are human pathogens.

Colonisation   The presence of an infectious agent in or on the body without causing injury or infection. It may persist indefinitely.

Commensal   A microorganism that lives on the body and benefits from being there whilst causing no harm to the host.

Contact   A person exposed to the risk of infection from being in close proximity to an infected person.

Contact bay   An area where contacts of a person known to be infected with or carrying an infection are nursed together to minimise the risk of spreading the infection to others who have not been exposed.

Contact tracing   Process of identifying contacts of an infected person.

Contamination

1. Transient presence of microorganisms in or on the body without causing injury or infection.
2. Not clean – soiled.
3. A contaminated sample has extraneous matter in it, e.g. skin flora in a blood culture sample.

COSHH   Control of substances hazardous to health.

Cross-infection   Infection of a person with microorganisms from another person.

Cumulative effect   Increasing antimicrobial effect associated with repeated application of a given antiseptic.

Cytostatic   Inhibits cell growth and division.

Cytotoxic   Toxic to cells.

Disinfection   The removal of most viable organisms using heat or chemicals (does not necessarily inactivate some viruses and bacterial spores).

Ectoparasite   A parasite that lives on the surface of the host.

EIA   Enzyme immunoassay – a test to detect antigens and antibodies. Often referred to as enzyme linked immunosorbent assays (ELISA).

Endemic   A persistent low or moderate level of disease in a population.

Endogenous infection   An infection where the source is thought to be the patient, e.g. MRSA in a wound in a patient known to carry MRSA on their skin.

Endoparasite   A parasite that lives inside the host.

Epidemic   An outbreak of an infectious disease that spreads rapidly and widely.

Exogenous infection   An infection where the source is thought to be external to the patient, i.e. transmitted from another source.

Exposure-prone procedure (EPP)   A procedure where there is a risk that injury to the healthcare worker may result in exposure of the patient's open tissues to the blood of the healthcare worker, e.g. where the healthcare worker's gloved hands are exposed to blades, needles and other sharp items inside the patient's open body cavity, wound or confined anatomical space where the hands or fingertips may not be fully visible at all times.

Fit testing   A series of movements carried out in a controlled setting whilst wearing an FFP3 mask to test how well it fits the wearer.

Fomites   Inanimate objects that can become contaminated and provide a vehicle for transmission of infection.
Herd immunity   Due to a high vaccine uptake there is reduced opportunity for a microorganism to be transmitted within a population.
Host   The person infected/infested with an organism.
Hyperendemic   A persistent high level of disease in a population.
Impedins   Factors that impede host defence mechanisms.
Incidence   The number of new cases of an infection over a given period of time.
Incubation period   The time when a person has been infected by an infectious agent but does not yet have clinical signs of infection.
Index case   The first person to have symptoms in an outbreak of infection.
Infection   Injury or invasion of the tissue caused by an infectious agent.
Infectious agent   The specific agent(s) causing the disease.
Infectious period   The time during which an infection can be passed from one person to another.
Infective dose   The number of microbes necessary to cause infection.
Inoculation injury   Sharps injury.
Invasiveness   The ability of an infectious agent to enter and spread in the body.
Liquor   Amniotic fluid.
Low-use outlet   A tap that is not used daily in augmented care areas or every three days in general areas.
Medical device   A product that has a medical use that is not medicine.
Mode of transmission   The mechanisms by which infectious agents are spread (direct contact, indirect, droplet and airborne).
Normal bacterial flora

Site	Normal flora
Mouth	Alpha-haemolytic streptococci
	Neisseria spp.
	Anaerobes
Nose, throat and sputum	Alpha-haemolytic streptococci
	Neisseria spp.
	Diphtheroids (Corynebacteria)
Skin	Coagulase-negative staphylococci
	Non-haemolytic streptococci
	Enterococci
	Diphtheroids (Corynebacteria) Propionibacteria
Bowel and faeces	Enterobacteriaceae (coliforms) Enterococci
	Anaerobes
	Candida
Vagina	Lactobacilli
	Alpha-haemolytic streptococci Diphtheroids (Corynebacteria)
	Group B streptococcus

Normal flora   The community of microorganisms that live on the human body.
Nosocomial   Hospital acquired.
Occurrence   Where the disease is known to occur and the population groups affected.
Opportunistic pathogen   A microorganism that would not normally cause disease under normal circumstances that is capable of causing disease when host defence mechanisms are impaired.

Outbreak   Two or more cases of the same infection that are linked, e.g. same ward/cared for by same healthcare worker/members of the same household, etc.

Pandemic   A global outbreak of an infectious disease.

Parasite   A parasite living in a close relationship with another organism (its host) and causing it harm.

Pathogen   A microorganism capable of causing disease.

Pathogenicity   The ability of a microorganism to cause disease.

PCR   Polymerase chain reaction – a test used to identify bacteria and viruses, quantify viral loads (the amount of virus in the bloodstream) and sometimes to test antibiotic sensitivities.

Period of infectivity/ communicability   Time when a person is shedding microorganisms and is infectious to others.

Personal protective equipment (PPE)   Gloves, aprons, gowns, masks and eye protection, which may be goggles or visors.

Post-exposure prophylaxis   Medicinal products given following a sharps/splash injury to prevent the injured person from developing a bloodborne virus infection.

PPM   Parts per million.

Prevalence   The total number of people with an infection over a given period of time.

Prophylaxis   Treatment given as a preventative measure.

Protective isolation   Nursing a person who is vulnerable to infection in a single room to protect them from transmission of infection.

Pyogenic   Pus forming.

Reservoir of infection   A permanent source of infection. This can be a person, an insect, an animal, a plant, a substance or an environment where an infectious agent can survive, live and multiply before transmission to a susceptible host.

Resident flora   Microorganisms residing under the superficial cells of the *stratum corneum* and also found on the surface of the skin.

Resistance   Mechanisms by which bacteria avoid destruction.

Respiratory hygiene   The practice of covering the mouth or nose when coughing or sneezing (using a tissue) followed by hand washing to prevent the spread of infection.

Screening   Taking of samples for microbiological testing to determine carriage of a microorganism in the absence of clinical signs of infection.

Sepsis   Clinical infection.

Septicaemia   The presence of an infectious agent in the blood with symptoms of infection.

Sharps injury   Needle prick, cut, scratch or bite injury.

Single use   Use item once and discard.

Single patient use   Item can be used more than once on same patient.

Source isolation   Nursing a person who has an infection in a single room to prevent transmission to others.

sp.   Species (singular).

Splash-generating procedure   An activity that creates a risk of splashing of blood or body fluids.

Splash injury   Blood/body fluid splash into the eyes, mouth or on to broken skin.

Sporadic   Occasional cases of a disease occurring at irregular intervals.

Spore   A tough protective coat that forms around a bacterial cell making it resistant to drying, heat and chemicals for months or even years.

spp.   Species (plural).

Sterilisation   The removal of all viable microorganisms, including viruses and bacterial spores.

Super-infection   When a person is infected with an infective agent and subsequently becomes infected with another infective agent at a later time.

Surveillance   Systematic process of observation, analysis and reporting of the incidence of disease in a population.

Susceptibility   Information on populations at risk of or resistant to infection/disease.

Susceptible host   A person at risk of infection/ disease.

Toxin   A substance released by a bacterial cell that causes ill effects within the body.

Transient flora (transient microbiota)   Microorganisms that colonise the superficial layers of the skin and are more amenable to removal by routine hand washing.

Vector   An organism that passes on a means of causing infection without becoming infected itself, e.g. mosquitoes are vectors in the transmission of malaria, as they carry the malarial parasites, which they inject into the host when they bite.

Vertical transmission   Transmission of infection from mother to child during pregnancy or childbirth.

Viral load   The number of viral particles in the blood used to measure disease progression or response to treatment.

Virulence   Characteristics of bacteria that enable them to cause infection and disease such as the ability to produce toxins, adhesins and impedins.

Visibly soiled hands.   Hands on which dirt or body fluids are readily visible.

Zoonoses   Diseases that can be passed from animals to humans.

6   Useful Resources

Aseptic Non-Touch Technique (ANTT)
http://www.antt.org.uk/ANTT_Site/Home.html

British Infection Association
http://www.britishinfection.org/drupal/

Care Quality Commission
www.cqc.org.uk

Central Sterilizing Club
www.csc.org.uk

Centres for Disease Control and Prevention
www.cdc.gov

Department of Health
http://www.dh.gov.uk/en/index.htm

Healthcare Infection Society
www.his.org.uk

Public Health England
http://www.gov.uk/government/organisations/public-health-england

Health Protection Scotland
www.hps.scot.nhs.uk

Infection Prevention Society
www.ips.uk.net

Institute of Public Health in Ireland
www.publichealth.ie

London Health Observatory
www.lho.org.uk

National Electronic Library of Infection
http://www.neli.org.uk/IntegratedCRD.nsf/NeLI_Home1?OpenForm

National Resource for Infection Control (Space for Health)
http://www.nric.org.uk/IntegratedCRD.nsf/NRIC_Home1?OpenForm

National Travel Health Network and Centre
http://www.nathnac.org/travel/index.htm

Public Health Wales
www.publichealthwales.wales.nhs.uk

World Health Organization
http://www.who.int/en/

Rapid Infection Control Nursing, First Edition. Shona Ross and Sarah Furrows.
© 2014 John Wiley & Sons, Ltd. Published 2014 by John Wiley & Sons, Ltd.

7 References, Sources and Further Reading

Advisory Committee on Dangerous Pathogens (2005) *Biological Agents: Managing the Risks in Laboratories and Healthcare Premises* [online] [07.01.13] http://www.hse.gov.uk/biosafety/biologagents.pdf

Advisory Committee on Dangerous Pathogens (May 2012) *Management of Hazard Group 4 Viral Haemorrhagic Fevers and Similar Human Infectious Diseases of High Consequence.* Department of Health, London.

Aseptic Non Touch Technique (2012) *The ANTT-Approach* [online] [30.01.13] http://www.antt.org.uk/ANTT_Site/ANTT-Approach.html

Ayliffe, G.A.J., Babb, J.R., Quoraishai, A.H. (1978) A test for 'hygienic' hand disinfection. *Journal of Clinical Pathology*, **31**(10), 923–928.

Barker, L.F. (1981) Pests in hospitals. *Journal of Hospital Infection*, **2**, 5–9.

British Medical Journal Group and Pharmaceutical Press (2012) Scabies. In *British National Formulary* [online] [25.11.12] http://www.medicinescomplete.com/mc/bnf/current/PHP8065-scabies.htm

Brittanica online encyclopedia (2013) *Asepsis* [online] [29.01.13] http://www.britannica.com/EBchecked/topic/38037/asepsis

Centers for Disease Control and Prevention (2013) *Prevention Strategies for Seasonal Influenza in Healthcare Settings: Guidelines and Recommendations* [online] [20.01.13] http://www.cdc.gov/flu/professionals/infectioncontrol/healthcaresettings.htm

Centers for Disease Control and Prevention (2012) *Group B Strep Infection in Adults* [online] [14.10.12] http://www.cdc.gov/groupbstrep/about/adults.html

Centers for Disease Control and Prevention (2010) *Prevention of Perinatal Group B Streptococcal Disease.* Morbidity and Mortality Weekly Report 2010; 59 (RR-10) [online] [14.10.12] http://www.cdc.gov/mmwr/pdf/rr/rr5910.pdf

Centers for Disease Control and Prevention (2007) *Guideline for Isolation Precautions: Preventing Transmission of Infectious Agents in Healthcare Settings.* Centers for Disease Control, Atlanta.

Coia, E., Duckworth, G.J., Edwards, D.I., *et al.* (2006) Guidelines for the control and prevention of methicillin-resistant *Staphylococcus aureus* (MRSA) in healthcare facilities. *Journal of Hospital Infections*, **66**(S1), 1–44. http://www.his.org.uk/_db/_documents/mrsa_guidelines_pdf.pdf

Crowcroft, N.S., Roth, C.E., Cohen, B.J., Miller, E.(1999) Guidance for control of parvovirus B19 infection in healthcare settings and the community. *Journal of Public Health Medicine*, **21**(4), 439–446. http://jpubhealth.oxfordjournals.org/content/21/4/439.full.pdf+html?ijkey=HU7938fXvuJ2g&keytype=ref&siteid=jphm

Curtis, G., Gemmell, D., Edwards, D.I., Fraise, A.P., *et al.* (2006) Guidelines for the prophylaxis and treatment of methicillin-resistant *Staphylococcus aureus* (MRSA) infections in the UK. *Journal of Antimicrobial Chemotherapy*, **57**(4), 589–608.

Department of Health (2002) *Hepatitis C Infected Healthcare Workers.* Department of Health, London.

Department of Health (2006) *Saving Lives: A Delivery Programme to Reduce Healthcare Associated Infection Including MRSA. High Impact Intervention No 6: Reducing the Risk of Infection from and the Presence of Clostridium difficile* [27.08.12] [online] http://www.dh.gov.uk/prod_consum_dh/groups/dh_digitalassets/@dh/@en/documents/digitalasset/dh_4135387.pdf

Department of Health (2007) *Saving Lives: A Delivery Programme to Reduce Healthcare Associated Infection Including MRSA.* Department of Health, London.

Rapid Infection Control Nursing, First Edition. Shona Ross and Sarah Furrows.
© 2014 John Wiley & Sons, Ltd. Published 2014 by John Wiley & Sons, Ltd.

Department of Health (2007) *Health Clearance for Tuberculosis, Hepatitis B, Hepatitis C and HIV: New Healthcare Workers*. Department of Health, London.

Department of Health (2007) *Hepatitis B Infected Healthcare Workers and Antiviral Therapy*. Department of Health, London.

Department of Health (2008) *The Health and Social Care Act 2008 (2010)*. Department of Health, London.

Department of Health (2009) *High Impact Intervention No 8: Care Bundle to Improve the Cleaning and Decontamination of Clinical Equipment*. Department of Health, London.

Department of Health (2010) *The Health and Social Care Act 2008: Code of Practice on the Prevention and Control of Infections and Related Guidance*. Department of Health, London.

Department of Health (2011) *Safe Management of Healthcare Waste Version: 2.0England* [online] [10.01.13] http://www.dh.gov.uk/prod_consum_dh/groups/dh_digitalassets/documents/digitalasset/dh_133874.pdf

Department of Health (2011) *Immunisation Against Infectious Disease* [online] [07.10.11] http://www.dh.gov.uk/prod_consum_dh/groups/dh_digitalassets/@dh/@en/documents/digitalasset/dh_130279.pdf

Department of Health (2012) *Water Sources and Potential Pseudomonas aeruginosa Contamination of Taps and Water Systems – Advice for Augmented Care Units* [online] http://www.dh.gov.uk/en/Publicationsandstatistics/Publications/PublicationsPolicyAndGuidance/DH_133317

Department of Health (2012) Haemophilus influenza type B (Hib). In *The Green Book* [online] [11.10.12] https://www.wp.dh.gov.uk/immunisation/files/2012/09/Green-Book-updated-280912.pdf

Department of Health (2012) Varicella. In *The Green Book* (online) [25.11.12] https://www.wp.dh.gov.uk/immunisation/files/2012/07/Green-Book-Chapter-34-v2_0.pdf

Department of Health/Advisory Committee on Antimicrobial Resistance and Healthcare Associated Infection (2011*)* *Antimicrobial Stewardship: Start Smart – Then Focus. Guidance for Antimicrobial Stewardship in Hospitals (England)* [online] [22.01.13] http://www.dh.gov.uk/prod_consum_dh/groups/dh_digitalassets/documents/digitalasset/dh_131181.pdf

Department of Health/Advisory Committee on Antimicrobial Resistance and Healthcare Associated Infection (2012) *Updated Guidance on the Diagnosis and Reporting of Clostridium difficile* [online] [07.10.12] http://www.dh.gov.uk/prod_consum_dh/groups/dh_digitalassets/@dh/@en/documents/digitalasset/dh_133016.pdf

Department of Health and Health Protection Agency (2008) *Clostridium difficile Infection: How to Deal with the Problem* [online] [27.08.12] http://www.hpa.org.uk/webc/HPAwebFile/HPAweb_C/1232006607827

Essex Health Protection Unit (2005) *Guidelines for the Prevention and Control of Infection in Essex Ambulance Service* [online] [11.11.09] http://www.hpa.org.uk/web/HPAwebFile/HPAweb_C/1194947372009

Essex Health Protection Unit (2009) *Factsheet on Biting Bugs* [online] [11.11.09] http://www.hpa.org.uk/web/HPAwebFile/HPAweb_C/1194947330183

Fraise, A.P., Bradley, C. (eds) (2009) *Ayliffe's Control of Healthcare-Associated Infection*. Hodder Arnold, London.

Hand Hygiene Task Force (2002) Guideline for hand hygiene in health-care settings. Recommendations of the Healthcare Infection Control Practices Advisory Committee and the HICPAC/SHEA/APIC/IDSA Hand Hygiene Task Force. *Morbidity and Mortality Weekly Report*, **51**(16), 1–48.

Hawker, J., Begg, N., Blair, I., Reintjes, R., Weinberg, J. (2001) *Communicable Disease Control Handbook*. Blackwell Science, Oxford.

Healing, T.D., Hoffman, P.N., Young, S.E.J. (1995) Communicable Disease Report: The infection hazards of human cadavers. *CDR Review*, **5**(5), R61–R68 [online] [19.01.13] http://www.hpa.org.uk/cdr/archives/CDRreview/1995/cdrr0595.pdf

Health and Safety Commission (1991) *Safety in Health Service Laboratories. Safe Working and the Prevention of Infection in Clinical Laboratories*. HMSO.

Health and Safety Executive (2005) *Biological Agents: Managing the Risks in Laboratories and Healthcare Premises* [online] [07.01.13] http://www.hse.gov.uk/biosafety/biologagents.pdf

Health and Safety Executive (2009) *Filtering Face Piece (FFP3) Masks* [online] [03.12.12] http://www.hse.gov.uk/news/2009/facemasks.htm

Health and Safety Executive (2013) *CE Marking* [online] [08.01.13] http://www.hse.gov.uk/work-equipment-machinery/ce-mark-summary.htm

Health and Safety Executive (2013) *CLP Regulation: Implications and Guidance* [online] [08.01.13] http://www.hse.gov.uk/ghs/implications.htm

Health and Safety Executive (2013) *What Is a 'Substance Hazardous to Health'?* [online] [08.01.12] http://www.hse.gov.uk/coshh/basics/substance.htm

Health and Safety Executive (2013) *What Is a Hazardous Substance* [online] [08.01.12] http://www.hse.gov.uk/coshh/detail/substances.htm

Health and Safety Executive (2013) *Zoonoses* [online] [13.01.13] http://www.hse.gov.uk/biosafety/diseases/zoonoses.htm

Health and Safety Executive (2013) *United Nations Globally Harmonised System of Classification and Labelling of Chemicals (GHS)* [online] [08.01.13] http://www.hse.gov.uk/ghs/index.htm

Health Protection Agency (2008) *Group B Streptococcal Infections – Frequently Asked Questions* [online] [14.10.12] http://www.hpa.org.uk/Topics/InfectiousDiseases/InfectionsAZ/StreptococciGroupB/General Information/strepGroupBFAQs/

Health Protection Agency (2008) *Guidance on the Diagnosis and Management of PVL-Associated Staphylococcus aureus Infections (PVL-SA) in England*. Health Protection Agency.

Health Protection Agency (2009) *Guidance for the Prevention and Control of Hepatitis A infection*. Health Protection Agency.

Health Protection Agency (2011) *Hepatitis C in the UK*, Report. Health Protection Agency.

Health Protection Agency (2011) *Guidance on Viral Rash in Pregnancy. Investigation, Diagnosis and Management of Viral Rash Illness, or Exposure to Viral Rash Illness, in Pregnancy* [online] http://www.hpa.org.uk/webc/HPAwebFile/HPAweb_C/1294740918985

Health Protection Agency (2011) *Chickenpox General Information* [online] [07.10.11] http://www.hpa.org.uk/Topics/InfectiousDiseases/InfectionsAZ/ChickenpoxVaricellaZoster/GeneralInformation/

Health Protection Agency (2011) *Factsheet on Biting Bugs* [online] [12.02.12] http://www.hpa.org.uk/webc/HPAwebFile/HPAweb_C/1194947330183

Health Protection Agency (2011) *English National Point Prevalence Survey on Healthcare-Associated Infections and Antimicrobial Use* [online] [22.01.13] http://www.hpa.org.uk/webc/HPAwebFile/HPAweb_C/1317134304594

Health Protection Agency (2012) *Public Health Management of Pertussis; HPA Guidelines for the Public Health Management of Pertussis Incidents in Healthcare Settings* [online] http://www.hpa.org.uk/webc/HPAwebFile/HPAweb_C/1317136713302

Health Protection Agency (2012) *Clostridium difficile* [online] [24.08.12] http://www.hpa.org.uk/Topics/InfectiousDiseases/InfectionsAZ/ClostridiumDifficile/

Health Protection Agency (2012) *Clostridium difficile: General Information* [online] [24.08.12] http://www.hpa.org.uk/Topics/InfectiousDiseases/InfectionsAZ/ClostridiumDifficile/GeneralInformation/

Health Protection Agency (2012) *HPA Guidelines for the Public Health Management of Pertussis* (updated October 2012) [online] http://www.hpa.org.uk/webc/HPAwebFile/HPAweb_C/1287142671506

Health Protection Agency (2012) *Essex Health Protection Unit Factsheet on Scabies* [online] 25.11.12] http://www.hpa.org.uk/webc/HPAwebFile/HPAweb_C/1194947413004

Health Protection Agency (2012) *General Information: Shingles* [online] [25.11.12] http://www.hpa.org.uk/Topics/InfectiousDiseases/InfectionsAZ/Shingles/GeneralInformationShingles/

Health Protection Agency (2012) *Infection Control Precautions during the Clinical Management of Drug Users with Possible, Probable or Confirmed Anthrax* [online] [22.01.13] http://www.hpa.org.uk/webc/HPAwebFile/HPAweb_C/1267549743963

Health Protection Agency (2012) *Infection Control Precautions to Minimise Transmission of Seasonal Influenza in the Healthcare Setting 2011–12* [online] [20.01.13] http://www.hpa.org.uk/webc/hpaweb-file/hpaweb_c/1317131892566

Health Protection Agency (2012) *List of Notifiable Diseases* [online] [20.01.13] http://www.hpa.org.uk/Topics/InfectiousDiseases/InfectionsAZ/NotificationsOfInfectiousDiseases/ListOfNotifiableDiseases/

Health Protection Agency (2012) *Local Services* [online] [20.01.13] http://www.hpa.org.uk/AboutTheHPA/WhoWeAre/LocalServices/

Health Protection Agency (2012) *Reporting Procedures* [online] [20.01.13] http://www.hpa.org.uk/Topics/InfectiousDiseases/InfectionsAZ/NotificationsOfInfectiousDiseases/ReportingProcedures/

Health Protection Agency and the Chartered Institute of Environmental Health (2012) *Public Health Operational Guidelines for Typhoid and Paratyphoid (Enteric Fever)*.

Health Protection Agency, Healthcare Infection Society, Infection Prevention Society, National Concern for Healthcare Infections, NHS Confederation (March 2012) *Guidelines for the Management of Norovirus*

Outbreaks in Acute and Community Health and Social Care Settings [online] http://www.hpa.org.uk/webw/HPAweb&HPAwebStandard/HPAweb_C/1317131647275

Health Protection Agency Regional Microbiology Network (2007) *A Good Practice Guide to Control Clostridium difficile* [27.08.12] [online] http://www.hpa.org.uk/web/HPAwebFile/HPAweb_C/1194947384014

Health Protection Scotland/NHS National Services Scotland (2012) *National Infection Prevention and Control Manual* [online] [04.12.12] http://www.documents.hps.scot.nhs.uk/hai/infection-control/ic-manual/ipcm-p-v1.0.pdf

Heaton, K.W., Radvan, J., Cripps, H., *et al.* (1992) Defeacation frequency and timing and stool form in the general population: a prospective study. *GUT*, **33**, 818–824.

Heymann, D.L. (ed) (2008) *Control of Communicable Diseases Manual*, 19th edition. American Public Health Association, Washington DC.

Infection Prevention Society (2011) *Quality Improvement Tool* [online] [22.01.13] http://www.ips.uk.net/template1.aspx?PageID=84&cid=91&category=Quality-Improvement-Tool

Johnson, A. (2007) *Johnson Outlines New Measures to Tackle Hospital Bugs* [online] [24.06.08] http://nds.coi.gov.uk/environment/mediaDetail.asp?MediaDetailsID=215726&NewsAreaID=2&ClientID=46&LocaleID=2

Lawrence, J., May, D. (2003) *Infection Control in the Community*. Churchill Livingstone, Edinburgh.

Medicines and Healthcare Regulatory Agency (2012) *Cryptic Clue or Familiar Sign?* [online] [27.11.12] http://www.mhra.gov.uk/home/groups/dts-bs/documents/publication/con076420.pdf

Medicines and Healthcare Regulatory Agency (2012) *Buying Medical Devices* [online] [23.01.13] http://www.mhra.gov.uk/Safetyinformation/Generalsafetyinformationandadvice/Adviceandinformationforconsumers/Buyingmedicaldevices/index.htm

Nathwani, D., Morgan, M., Masterton, R.G., Dryden, M., Cookson, B.D., French, G., Lewis, D. (2008) Guidelines for UK practice for the diagnosis and management of methicillin-resistant *Staphylococcus aureus* (MRSA) infections presenting in the community. *Journal of Antimicrobial Chemotherapy*, **61**, 976–994. http://jac.oxfordjournals.org/content/61/5/976.full.pdf

National Institute of Clinical Excellence (2002) *Principles for Best Practice in Clinical Audit* [online] [29.01.13] http://www.nice.org.uk/niceMedia/pdf/BestPracticeClinicalAudit.pdf

National Institute for Clinical Excellence (2003) *Infection Control: Prevention of Healthcare-Associated Infections in Primary and Community Care* [online] www.nice.org.uk/pdf/Infection

National Patient Safety Agency (2004) *Clean Your Hands Campaign*. NPSA, London. www.npsa.nhs.uk

National Patient Safety Agency (2007) *Safer Practice Notice 15: Colour Coding Hospital Cleaning Materials and Equipment* [online] [11.01.07] http://www.npsa.nhs.uk/site/media/documents/2140_0429colourcodingsp1D2F4.pdf

National Patient Safety Agency (2008) *Patient Safety Alert – Clean Hands Save Lives*, 2nd edition. NPSA, London. www.npsa.nhs.uk

National Patient Safety Agency National Reporting and Learning Service (2009) *The Revised Healthcare Cleaning Manual* [online] [21.01.13] http://www.nrls.npsa.nhs.uk/EasySiteWeb/getresource.axd?AssetID=61814&type=full&servicetype=Attachment

Newcastle Hospitals (2009) *Animals in Hospital Policy* [online] [27.05.10] http://www.newcastlehospitals.org.uk/downloads/policies/Health%20and%20Safety/AnimalsonHospitalPremises200907.pdf

NHS ESTATES (2002) *Infection Control in the Built Environment*. The Stationery Office, London.

NICE (March 2011) *Clinical Diagnosis and Management of Tuberculosis, and Measures for its Prevention and Control. NICE Clinical Guideline* [online] http://guidance.nice.org.uk/CG117

Pratt, R.J., Pellowe, C.M., Wilson, J.A., Loveday, H.P., Harper, P.J., Jones, S.R.L.J., McDougall, C., Wilcox, M.H. (2007) Epic2: National evidence-based guidelines for preventing healthcare-associated infections in NHS hospitals in England. *The Journal of Hospital Infection*, **65S**, S1–S64.

Prescott, L.M., Harley, J.P., Klein, D.A. (2002) *Microbiology*, 5th edition. McGraw-Hill, New York.

Rowley, S., Clare, S. (2009) *Improving Standards of Aseptic Practice Through an ANTT Trust-wide Implementation Process: A Matter of Prioritisation and Care* [online] [26.0.13] http://bji.sagepub.com/content/10/1_suppl/s18

Rowley, S., Clare, S. (2011) *ANTT: A Standard Approach to Aseptic Technique* [online] [29.01.13] http://www.nursingtimes.net/Journals/2011/09/09/s/z/e/130911_review_Rowley.pdf

Rowley, S., Sinclair, S. (2004) *Working Towards an NHS Standard for Aseptic Non-touch Technique* [online] [29.01.13] http://www.nursingtimes.net/Journals/2012/11/23/d/h/s/040224SuppANTT.pdf

Royal College of Nursing (2013) *Chapter Three: Transcultural Nursing Care of Adults* [online] [30.01.13] http://www.rcn.org.uk/development/learning/transcultural health/transcultural/adulthealth/ sectionthree

. Royal Society for the Prevention of Cruelty to Animals (2012) *Keep Fleas in Check* [online] [12.02.12] http://www.rspca.org.uk/allaboutanimals/pets/general/fleas

Sax, H., Allegranzi, B., Uçkay, I., Larson, E., Boyce, J., Pittet, D. (2007) 'My five moments for hand hygiene': a user-centred design approach to understand, train, monitor and report hand hygiene. *The Journal of Hospital Infection*, **67**, 9–21.

Sleigh J.D., Timbury M.C. (1998) *Notes on Medical Bacteriology*, 5th edition. Churchill Livingstone, Edinburgh.

South Cambridgeshire District Council (2012) *Fleas* [online] [12.02.12] http://www.scambs.gov.uk/ environment/pestsandnuisance/insectpests/fleas.htm

Spicer, W.J. (2000) *Clinical Bacteriology*, Mycology and Parasitology. Churchill Livingstone, London.

The National Archives (2012) *HCAI: Reducing Healthcare Associated Infections* [online] [27.01.13] http:// webarchive.nationalarchives.gov.uk/20120118164404/http://hcai.dh.gov.uk/whatdoido/high-impact-interventions/

UK Health Departments (1998) *Guidance for Clinical Health Care Workers: Protection Against Infection with Blood-borne Viruses. Recommendations of the Expert Advisory Group on AIDS and the Advisory Group on Hepatitis.* Department of Health, Wetherby.

United Nations (2011) *Globally Harmonized System of Classification and Labeling of Chemicals*, 4th edition [online] [08.01.13] http://www.unece.org/fileadmin/DAM/trans/danger/publi/ghs/ghs_rev04/ English/ST-SG-AC10-30-Rev4e.pdf

Viral Gastroenteritis Subcommittee of the Scientific Advisory Committee of the National Disease Surveillance Centre (2003) *National Guidelines on The Management of Outbreaks of Norovirus Infection in Healthcare Settings.* National Disease Surveillance Centre, Dublin.

Wilson, J. (2001) *Infection Control in Clinical Practice*, 2nd edition. Bailliere Tindal, London.

Woodhead, K., Taylor, E.W., Bannister, G., Chesworth, T., Hoffman, P., Humphreys, H. (Hospital Infection Society Working Party) (2002) *Behaviours and Rituals in the Operating Theatre* [online] [21.12.12] http://www.his.org.uk/_db/_documents/Rituals-02.pdf

World Health Organisation (2009) *WHO Guidelines on Hand Hygiene in Health Care* [online] [26.11.12] http://whqlibdoc.who.int/publications/2009/9789241597906_eng.pdf

Index

Page numbers in *italics* denote figures, those in **bold** denote tables.

Rapid Infection Control Nursing, First Edition. Shona Ross and Sarah Furrows.
© 2014 John Wiley & Sons, Ltd. Published 2014 by John Wiley & Sons, Ltd.

Printed and bound by CPI Group (UK) Ltd, Croydon, CR0 4YY

Printed and bound by CPI Group (UK) Ltd, Croydon, CR0 4YY

09/10/2024

14571429-0002